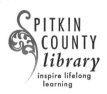

JEN SWEENEY

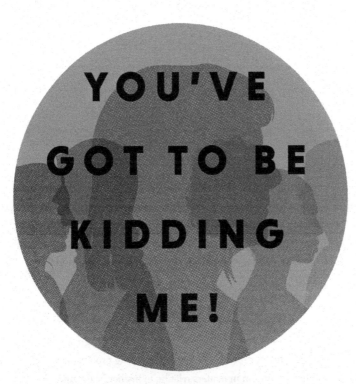

YOU'VE
GOT TO BE
KIDDING
ME!

PERIMENOPAUSE
Symptoms, Stages,
and Strategies

Print ISBN: 978-1-66782-765-0
eBook ISBN: 978-1-66782-766-7

This book is solely for the purpose of education and personal growth. It should not be used as a substitute for medical advice from medical professionals. The reader should consult a clinician in matters relating to his/her health and fitness and particularly with respect to any symptoms that may require diagnosis or medical attention. In the event of physical or mental distress, please consult with an appropriate medical professional. Consult a health professional before performing any exercise program. It is your responsibility to evaluate your own medical and physical condition and to independently determine whether to perform, use or adapt any of the information or content in this book.

This book is a product of Periwinkle Group LLC. The author of this book and Periwinkle Group LLC disclaim liability for any loss or damage suffered by any person as a result of the information or content in this book. The information in this book is for educational and personal growth purposes only.

This guide is dedicated to my daughter, Hadley, and to her peers.

May they and all future generations of girls and women have access to information and

health-care services that help them care for their bodies and thrive.

May they live in cultures that respect their reproductive and sexual health.

TABLE OF CONTENTS

WELCOME!

Welcome, I'm so glad you are here!

THIS GUIDE IS FOR YOU

This guide is for you and every woman out there who wants to be ready for perimenopause. My hope in writing this guide is that it will give you invaluable information to prepare for perimenopause, the transition to menopause when our bodies begin to make fewer hormones. Perimenopause is a stage of life that can last for fifteen years for some women, so we need to be prepared. Alongside the in-depth research featured throughout the book are personal anecdotes and quotes from women who have gone through perimenopause and not only made it to the other side, but are happy, healthy and thriving. I also share a lot about my own perimenopause journey with the hope that what I experienced can help others.

My greatest hope is that you—and all women—sail through perimenopause with little to no symptoms or changes to your life. The reality, though, is that perimenopause can be a very destabilizing and challenging time for many of us and there is no way to predict how you will be affected. It's very important to prepare *now* in case—like me—you are hit with a tsunami of symptoms that put your career, friendships and intimate relationships at risk.

Most of us are told very little about what to expect in perimeno-pause, menopause and beyond. Many of us live in cultures that consider women's sexual and reproductive issues taboo or uncomfortable to talk about[1]. Very, very few women I have spoken with have talked with their own mothers and aunts about what to expect as we age. Several years ago, I was at a girls' night out and I learned that most of my friends were pretty much in the dark about anything beyond birth control and mammograms. Your friends likely don't have a clue either and can't help themselves let alone help you! That's why I created this guide. We shouldn't be fumbling around in the dark trying to find answers to a natural stage in women's lives. It's 2021 as I write this guide and it's time we had more information available to us.

It's not just the lack of information that's a problem. It's also that perimenopause in some ways sneaks up on us and for some of us it wreaks havoc physically and emotionally. In our late teens and twenties we're focused on getting an education. Then we work hard to secure a job or launch a career. Lots of us become mothers and our children and families constantly pull us in a million different directions. I was so busy in my thirties the last thing I had time for was thinking about my own health. I don't advise that, by the way!

My point is that many of us spend our early adult years putting everything and everyone ahead of ourselves and our own needs. We ignore our health, we forget our bodies will evolve and we don't prepare ourselves for what's to come. Some of us forget we even have needs! I'm glad you found this guide because you deserve to take the time to understand what may lie ahead for your health and well-being. This guide is for every woman who is curious and maybe even a little scared

---

1   Lisa Selin Davis, "The $10 Billion Business of Perimenopause." *Fast Company*, April 2021.

about what's ahead. It's for all of you who want to be prepared, who want to hear from other women about their experiences and who want to know you aren't alone in this journey. Not only aren't you alone, more than 1 billion women around the world will have experienced perimenopause by 2025.[2] Welcome, welcome, welcome. I'm so glad you're here.

WHAT THIS GUIDE *IS*

This guide *is* easy to read and chock-full of information you'll relate to. I wrote it in this way so you can digest it swiftly and become an advocate for yourself as quickly as possible.

This guide *is* "quick and dirty." In other words, I read all the books, did all the research and took all the notes so you don't have to. Let's be real: you don't have time for that! I went through the research with a fine-tooth comb to create a guide that gives you the most important information you need to know to thrive during perimeno-pause. Quick and dirty!

This guide *is* the beginning of a journey in which you have the information, the peer support and the skills you need to experience your perimenopause years with as much joy and laughter as possible. Join us at www.helloperiwinkle.com for in-depth courses on various women's health issues, personal stories from women, an online support community and our *Peri Lab*, where we will test and share reviews on perimenopause products.

This guide includes composite stories and quotes based on inter-views, surveys and conversations I had with women who are pre-per-imenopausal, in perimenopause and in menopause. These composite

---

2   Jessica Grose, "Why is Perimenopause Still Such a Mystery?," *New York Times*, April 2019,

stories and quotes are also based on interactions and friendships I formed in private thyroid and perimenopause groups. I chose to construct these composite stories to protect the confidence of the women who so openly shared with me. I also created these composite identities because in them I can reflect the wide diversity of experiences women shared with me versus a narrow set of individual experiences. With all of that said, the stories and quotes in this guide reflect women's true experiences: the good, the bad and the ugly.

WHAT THIS GUIDE IS *NOT*

This guide is *not* a be all, end all encyclopedia with every single thing a person could ever want to know about perimenopause. That would be way too long and no one has time for that!

This guide is *not* a medical document in any way, shape or form. I'm pretty sure no one thought that, but it's good to have down on paper! I am *not* a clinician and have no medical training. With that said, I *have* been a patient advocate for nearly two decades, and I have many years of experience researching and writing in the health-care field. Dr. Lakeischa McMillan was kind enough to read this guide prior to release to ensure the content is clinically accurate.

This guide is *not* a stand-alone guide if you don't want it to be. Periwinkle's (www.helloperiwinkle.com) goal is to create in-depth courses and other kinds of engaging content on specific issues that matter to you about perimenopause, middle age and more. Join us there to continue the conversation and the journey—together!

Let's dive in!

Chapter 1:

_____

WHY I NEEDED THIS GUIDE FOUR YEARS AGO

This guide is a cautionary tale—my cautionary tale! I wrote it because I don't want other women to experience the difficulties I did with perimenopause. In my early forties I was fit, strong and happy. I had a great relationship with my husband, including a fulfilling sex life, and I had just founded a successful business that brought me a great deal of satisfaction. My life brought me a tremendous amount of joy and laughter and I was incredibly grateful.

The thing about perimenopause is that it flies under the radar. Our society, including many health-care providers, doesn't talk about it the way we discuss pregnancy, for example. In fact, you may have never even heard the term before you picked up this guide. Many of the women I spoke to during the research process told me the word was completely novel to them.

I was in my mid-forties when perimenopause snuck up on me. I began to feel tired all the time. This was not your "I missed a night of sleep" tired. I was exhausted deep down into my bones.

My lack of energy was problematic because I had two teenagers at home, three dogs (yes, we're crazy), an active social life, a husband I loved and I wanted to spend time with, community responsibilities and a company to run. I spent each and every day disappointed in myself for not getting through my lengthy to-do lists. The things I wasn't able to get done kept piling up and I started to worry I would never get back to the person I used to be: "a get sh$t done-er."

I became riddled with anxiety. Anxiety runs in my family so I was very familiar with it and I had experienced it as a teenager and in my twenties. But, in my thirties I had tackled and tamed my anxiety. I realized exercise was the antidote so I made consistent exercise a core part of my life. I also discovered transcendental meditation and mindfulness, which both gave me a sense of peace about life. The truth was that anxiety hadn't been a part of my life for nearly fifteen years. It was back with a vengeance. I would awaken at four o'clock most mornings with a rapidly beating heart and a swirling brain ruminating on every possible thing in my life, unable to go back to sleep. I started having panic attacks and became nervous about performing at work. I was miserable.

Life only got worse as I found myself struggling through workouts, gaining weight despite healthy eating and finding more cellulite every time I looked in the mirror. I felt like my body was falling apart. Even the personal trainer I worked out with multiple times a week expressed concern. Neither of us could understand why I was struggling to build muscle, why I was gaining more and more weight and why I was in such pain in between workouts. To add to my misery—and to my husband's dismay—my sex drive completely tanked. My periods had become so heavy and my PMS so extreme that I was out of commission for a good week and a half out of every month.

Things came to a head one summer when I arrived home from a trip to Barnes & Noble and realized I had been walking all over the store for an hour with a huge bloodstain on the back of a pair of cute pink shorts. I was humiliated and I was also becoming depressed. When I looked at my life I knew I had much to be grateful for. I was at the top of my career. I had a loving family and great friends. But you can only go on for so long being exhausted and in pain before your mood is affected, and I was struggling to find anything to feel good about. I knew I had to do something.

This is the part of the story where things got frustrating and sad for me. In a couple of short years my health and well-being had declined to such a degree that I was certain I had a serious disease. In fact, I told my business partners and my husband I would likely need to stop working because things had gotten so bad. The hardest part was that I was completely alone in my painful journey. I went to several doctors but none of them seemed very concerned about what I was experiencing. One or two insinuated that women started experiencing health issues as they aged, but no one mentioned perimenopause. Perimenopause was also not something my girlfriends were talking about. My mother had never mentioned it either. I felt like I had arrived on a whole new planet, alone and, frankly, lonely, with no resources. The only things I had left were hope and determination.

Trying to solve a puzzle when you're exhausted, your mood is depressed and your body hurts is very difficult, but that's what I had to do. I climbed into my bed with every book I could find and read them closely, taking notes along the way. I spent months and months online reading medical journals and articles and I sought out alternative health-care providers in a search for a solution. The good news is that my efforts paid off. I learned a tremendous amount from my research. I didn't become a medical expert, but I knew far more than

7

I had when I started. I used my newfound knowledge to advocate for what I needed, and four years later I have my life back. I'm fit, healthy and happy. The company I built is thriving and my relationships are better than they've ever been.

Entering perimenopause was the most difficult time in my life. I swore to myself that if I was able to take back control of my body and spirit, I would share what I learned with as many people as possible to save them the same heartache. That's what this guide is: my gift to you. During my journey I learned some very important things:

Perimenopause is a significant stage in women's lives but is not fully understood by the medical community.

- Few resources are available to women as they enter perimenopause.

- There is little awareness among women about perimenopause and what it entails.

- Little emotional support is available to us as we navigate the perimenopause stage of our lives.

This book is just one part of Periwinkle, a movement I'm launching along with this guide. At Periwinkle we are:

- Raising awareness about perimenopause.

- Sharing information with women to help them advocate for themselves.

- Helping the medical community evolve in how it cares for women in perimenopause.

- Supporting women emotionally during perimenopause.

- Exploring ways clinicians and patients can work together to flip the script on perimenopause.

Periwinkle isn't just about perimenopause. It's about women in midlife. Many of us will have a good thirty to forty years ahead of us once we end perimenopause and enter menopause. Periwinkle isn't about midlife crises. It's about an open runway and the many horizons ahead of us to explore spiritually, emotionally, relationally and physically. Let's do amazing things together!

I hope you'll join me at www.helloperiwinkle.com and on our social media pages at:

Facebook: www.facebook.com/We-Are-Periwinkle-105879768567382

Instagram: @WeArePeriwinkle

TikTok: tiktok.com/@weareperiwinkle

Chapter 2:

WE ARE OUR OWN BEST HOPE

"**I WAS AT MY ANNUAL PHYSICAL. I WAS** thirty-eight years old, and I asked my doctor what to expect from perimenopause and menopause. He said: 'I'll tell you when you get there.' I felt so dismissed. Here I was trying to better understand what to expect in the same way I had done when I was pregnant and I was blown off." — *Neena*

If you're reading this guide it's likely you or someone you love is approaching perimenopause or in it currently. I commend you for preparing yourself for the journey ahead and for doing what you can to understand what you are undergoing right now physically and emotionally. The reality is that we know our bodies better than anyone else, including our clinicians, so it's important that we become knowledgeable and prepared for this stage of life. However, as you'll learn in what follows, the sad truth is that we must ready ourselves for perimenopause because it's highly unlikely anyone else will give us the information or resources we need. We are truly our own best hope when it comes to perimenopause.

Why is it important for us to be prepared for perimenopause? The bottom line is that perimenopause is a significant stage in women's lives. During perimenopause, our bodies are under a significant amount of stress that affects us physically, emotionally and mentally. Not only are we under stress due to perimenopause but many of us go through perimenopause just as we're hitting our peak earning years, while we're trying to launch teenagers off to college or to their first jobs and caring for elderly or sick parents.

Not only is perimenopause a significant stage in women's lives, but millions of women experience perimenopause every year. 1.3 million women enter menopause annually and every single one of them went through perimenopause prior to menopause.[3] Keep in mind that millennials are the largest generation in the workforce and the oldest millennials at thirty-nine are entering the perimenopausal period.

Perimenopause and menopause are not just stages in a woman's life that happen to have uncomfortable symptoms. Perimenopause and menopause, in particular, mean we are at greater risk for certain health issues. For example, hormonal changes can result in an accelerated increase in LDL cholesterol, which puts us at greater risk for heart disease. While loss of bone density occurs in both men and women as we age, for some women that loss is extreme due to plummeting levels of estrogen. This puts them at greater risk of osteoporosis and broken bones.

One 2017 study found that the more severe and longer lasting a woman's hot flashes and night sweats are, the greater her risk for

---

3   www.ncbi.nlm.nih.gov/books/NBK507826

developing type 2 diabetes.[4] Perimenopause and menopause are signs our bodies are aging and when we are properly treated for the symptoms we experience, we're not just treating uncomfortable symptoms. We're taking steps that can lower our risk for diseases in the last third of our lives, so why isn't more information available about perimenopause? Keep reading.

I run a purpose-driven health-care consulting company called X4 Health (www.x4health.com) with two other women cofounders. I have spent twenty years in the health-care field and I have developed deep expertise in many health-care issues despite not being a clinician. Prior to founding X4 Health, I was a patient advocate and fought for many decades to make the health-care industry a place in which patients' and families' needs were prioritized. All of these years later, I'm very proud of that work and the changes I achieved. Yet, even with my background, my perimenopause experience was a serious wake-up call! It reminded me the health-care industry is a very, very long way from meeting women's needs.

This may come as a shock to you, but the vast majority of clinicians receive *no* training in medical school or in residency focused on women's health after their reproductive years. According to a study by researchers at Johns Hopkins, only 20 percent of residency programs have a formal menopause curriculum.[5] Most family medicine, internal medicine and—get this—OB/GYN residency programs include at

---

4   The North American Menopause Society (NAMS). "Hot flashes could be precursor to diabetes, study suggests: Data demonstrates effect of severity and duration of hot flashes on risk of developing diabetes." ScienceDaily. www.sciencedaily.com/releases/2017/12/171206090537.htm

5   Christianson MS, Ducie JA, Altman K, Khafagy AM, Shen W. Menopause education: Needs assessment of American obstetrics and gynecology residents. *Menopause.* 2013 Nov;20(11):1120–1125. doi: 10.1097/GME.0b013e31828ced7f. PMID: 23632655.

most one hour of instruction on menopause. Things get worse when it comes to perimenopause. My team and I did a tremendous amount of research, yet we were unable to unearth any medical curricula that address perimenopause. None.

Unfortunately, the health-care system and many practitioners themselves are way behind. Until I sought help specifically for perimenopause, not one of my doctors spoke with me about perimenopause or shared with me the symptoms for which I should be on the lookout. Even worse, when I raised my symptoms with some doctors, they waved off my concerns with blanket statements like: "Aging is hard, but it happens to the best of us," and, "Well, I wouldn't recommend hormone treatments. There's lots of problems with them."

Let me be clear: I have *deep admiration* for clinicians and I know the vast majority have gone into health care because they care about patients and want to make a difference in people's lives. However, the hard truth is most clinicians are woefully lacking in training on women's health. In 2022, women's health is still considered puberty, pregnancy and postpartum. What about the estimated 38 million American women who are menopausal and who account for approximately 20 percent of the American workforce? What about those same women who go through perimenopause before they get to menopause? That's a lot of women whose needs are *not* being met. Worse than that, many of their needs are not even acknowledged!

It's important we have access to information *before* we are in perimenopause so we can be on the lookout for symptoms, prepare ourselves should we experience physical, emotional and mental changes and make sure we have support available to us. The good news is that this guide includes the most up-to-date information you need to be your own best advocate. Information alone is not enough, so here is some additional advice to help you get the best care possible.

1. **Find a clinician who specializes in hormones.** While most of the health-care industry still doesn't address perimenopause, a growing number of practices and individual clinicians are focused on helping women balance their hormones and manage their symptoms. They are who you want to work with in perimenopause and ultimately menopause. I dive more deeply into this topic in Chapter 8.

2. **View yourself as a central part of your care team.** Please only work with clinicians who partner with you as a central part of the care team. Remember: you know your body better than anyone else ever could, including clinicians.

3. **Track your well-being.** Many of us are busy working, caring for our families and volunteering in our communities. We have put ourselves last, or at least near the bottom, for a long time. As a result, we may not have all the data we need to share with our clinicians. It's very important we have information about how often we have our periods and for how long, how long and well we are sleeping, our energy levels throughout the day, if and/or how often sex is uncomfortable etc. Collecting these data will give you and your care team a full picture of your health and well-being. You can find a great and comprehensive "Well-Being Tracker" on the Periwinkle website at www.hello-periwinkle.com/tracker

4. **Power through any shame or embarrassment.** Many of us have grown up in cultures that avoided talking about any women's health or reproduction issues. For some of us, those issues were not just avoided. They were also taboo or shameful. It can be difficult for many of us to talk with clinicians about personal issues, but when we hold information back, it

prevents our care team from being able to help us. If you feel unable to share with your care team fully, bring your Well-Being Tracker with you to appointments and that will help you give your care team the information they need to support you.

5. **Inquire about low-cost options.** My perimenopause experience has been expensive and you'll learn more about why that is in upcoming chapters, but in the meantime, keep in mind that we all deserve to feel better no matter our income or access to health insurance. Nutrition and supplements are for many of us key to improving our perimenopause experience, so make sure to explore those options with your care team as well.

6. **Take care of your emotional and mental well-being, not just your body.** For whatever reason, most of our health-care system separates physical well-being from emotional and mental well-being despite the fact that they're interconnected. Talk with your care team about challenges you may be experiencing, from anxiety to depression, as they could stem from physical changes and your health-care providers may have recommendations for managing those conditions. I talk more about this in Chapter 13.

Some of you may feel excited and look forward to feeling more empowered when you're done reading this guide. Others may feel overwhelmed. I get it. None of us need another thing on our overflowing plates! Don't worry; stick with me. I promise the time you spend with this guide will pay off. You'll feel better physically, and you'll be empowered by knowing and understanding what is happening to you and your body. Remember: *You* are central to your perimenopause journey.

Chapter 3:

_____

WHAT ARE THE STAGES AND SYMPTOMS OF PERIMENOPAUSE ANYWAY?

"AS I ENTERED MY MID-FORTIES, MY PERIODS went from a monthly, manageable inconvenience to something I dreaded. While I had always had cramps, suddenly they were borderline debilitating and on top of that, my periods were incredibly heavy. I spent at least a week of every month tearful with moments of rage. And, that was before the hot flashes and mgraines started! Miserable is the way I would describe those years." — *Jennie*

In many ways, women's health feels like a puzzle. It's not studied enough and clinicians don't receive adequate training focused on it. These issues are exacerbated by the fact that our culture doesn't embrace discussions about women's health, particularly for women in middle age and older.

For example, recently I heard a radio advertisement for a local hospital during which the announcer said: "We're here for you in pregnancy, in childbirth and later on with all the changes you may experience." I asked myself, "Later on? What does that mean? Changes? What changes?" I searched the hospital's website and couldn't find anything beyond pregnancy and childbirth except bone density scanning for osteoporosis (which is important, by the way). It's almost as though women's health needs disappear and we become invisible after we've had children or when we enter middle age.

This lack of understanding and of transparent information leads to many of us being unaware and at best confused about the health stages that await us after age thirty-five. Let's break it down because the best way for you to be an advocate of your own health and well-being is to understand these stages, including terminology and typical symptoms.

WOMEN'S MIDLIFE REPRODUCTIVE HEALTH STAGES

I. Perimenopause Stage

What is perimenopause?

- Perimenopause is the gradual transition toward menopause. The transition to menopause is a time during which our ovaries gradually produce less estrogen and other hormones.

  Note: People sometimes use the terms *premenopause* and *perimenopause* interchangeably, but premenopause is not a scientifically accepted term.

When does perimenopause begin?

- For many women, perimenopause begins in our forties. For a small percentage of women, the transition to perimenopause begins in their thirties.

How long does perimenopause last?

- For many women, perimenopause is an eight- to ten-year phase. Reread that sentence, please. It's important to understand that for many of us, perimenopause lasts a long time. A small portion of women begin perimenopause early and for them, the stage can last up to fifteen years. For others, perimenopause may only last two years, and a small percentage of women do not experience perimenopause at all. The average length of perimenopause is four years.[6]

How do you know you're in perimenopause?

- There is tremendous variability in when perimenopause begins and how long it lasts. There are two chief ways to know you're in perimenopause: tracking your symptoms and testing your hormones. I discuss both in great detail in the next couple of chapters.

How do you know perimenopause is over?

- Our ovaries release eggs for fertilization with the help of estrogen. When an egg is fertilized we become pregnant, and when an egg is not fertilized we get our menstrual period. In the last one to two years of perimenopause, the drop in our estrogen levels accelerates and we release fewer and fewer eggs for fertilization. The perimenopause stage

---

6   Harvard Health Publishing. *"Perimenopause: Rocky Road to Menopause."* Updated August 24, 2018. https://www.health.harvard.edu/womens-health/perimenopause-rocky-road-to-menopause

ends when our ovaries stop releasing eggs. For the vast majority of us, the end of perimenopause coincides with the conclusion of our monthly periods.

II. Menopause Stage

- Women begin to transition from perimenopause to menopause with erratic menstrual periods. When our menstrual periods end it means our ovaries have stopped releasing eggs for fertilization and we stop producing estrogen. Menopause is complete when we have gone without a menstrual period for a full year—twelve consecutive months.

- 1.3 million women in the United States alone enter menopause every year. This happens at age fifty-one on average, while 5 percent of women are menopausal by age forty-five.[7]

- When we go through menopause tends to be genetic and is unaffected by race, socioeconomic status or the age we began our period. Some of us go through menopause earlier than others due to lifestyle. For example, women who smoke start transitioning to menopause earlier. Other women go through menopause earlier if they have surgery on their ovaries or have a hysterectomy.[8]

---

7 www.ncbi.nlm.nih.gov/books/NBK507826

8 Siddle N, Sarrel P, Whitehead M. The effect of hysterectomy on the age at ovarian failure: Identification of a subgroup of women with premature loss of ovarian function and literature review. *Fertil Steril.* 1987;47:94–100.

- One percent of women enter early menopause (which can occur due to chemotherapy or hysterectomy) by age forty.[9]

III. Postmenopause Stage

- Postmenopause is the period of time (the rest of your life) after menopause. It is the name given to the period of time after a woman has not had a period for an entire year, although most people just continue to say "menopause".

WHAT TO LOOK OUT FOR: SIGNS AND SYMPTOMS OF PERIMENOPAUSE AND BEYOND

One of the chief reasons I wrote this book is so women know what to look for when it comes to perimenopause. When we begin menstruating, we know because we begin bleeding—usually monthly. Perimenopause, on the other hand, is different in that the symptoms don't begin overnight and they vary for women.

When we don't know what to look for, we can mistake the symptoms for other things, which means a delay in getting treatment or support. When I entered perimenopause, I felt like I had been hit by a Mack truck and I blamed myself. I told myself I was too stressed, not eating well enough, not sleeping enough.

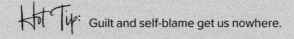 Hot Tip: Guilt and self-blame get us nowhere.

9   Luborsky JL, Meyer P, Sowers MF, Gold EB, Santoro N. Premature menopause in a multi-ethnic population study of the menopause transition. *Hum Reprod.* 2003;18:199–206.

In perimenopause the rate at which our ovaries produce estrogen begins to decrease. Not only does our body need to adjust to functioning with less estrogen but decreased estrogen disrupts the very important balance among estrogen, testosterone and progesterone, which I talk about in lots more detail in the next chapter. Not surprisingly, our body responds to these changes with what I call in this book *signs and symptoms*.

Not only do the signs and symptoms of perimenopause vary among women, women experience these signs and symptoms at a variety of ages. With that said, it's important to understand what you may experience so you recognize these symptoms if or when they do arise.

I. **Most Common Signs and Symptoms of Perimenopause**

- **Hot Flashes and Night Sweats.** More than 50 percent of perimenopausal women experience sudden increases in body temperature.[10] We sweat and feel flushed for about five to ten minutes. This often occurs at night but can also happen during the day. Hot flashes usually begin in the scalp, face, neck or chest. We all experience them differently. Some of us feel only slightly warm, while others of us end up wringing wet. Many women are confused when they begin experiencing hot flashes in their early forties as they associate them only with menopause, but *hot flashes are actually one of the most common symptoms of perimenopause.*

- **Irregular or Longer or Shorter Periods.** Before perimenopause our estrogen and progesterone levels rise and fall in a consistent pattern during our menstrual cycles.

---

10   Dalal, Pronob K, and Manu Agarwal. "Postmenopausal syndrome." *Indian Journal of Psychiatry* vol. 57, Suppl 2 (2015): S222–32. doi:10.4103/0019-5545.161483

In perimenopause hormone levels become more erratic, which can lead to unpredictable periods. Because our estrogen levels are dropping in perimenopause, our uterine lining becomes thinner, which means our periods may last for fewer days. Short cycles are more common in the earlier stages of perimenopause. Your whole cycle may also last two or three weeks instead of four. Many of us who are in perimenopause feel like our period just ended when the next one arrives. When we get further into perimenopause, our cycles may become much longer (more than thirty-eight days) and farther apart. This is because we are experiencing anovulatory cycles, meaning we are having a menstrual cycle without ovulation.

- **Heavier Periods.** On the other hand, we may experience heavier periods during perimenopause if our estrogen levels are higher than our progesterone levels. As early as our late thirties we start producing less progesterone. With less progesterone to regulate the growth of the endometrium, the uterine lining may become thicker before it is shed. If the estrogen levels have not decreased as much as the progesterone levels and are higher than they are, the uterine lining will thicken and result in heavier bleeding. Heavy bleeding is also called menorrhagia and it usually means you lose 80 mL or more blood during your period. You can assume you're experiencing heavy periods if you're bleeding through your tampon, menstrual cup or pad quickly.

- **Worsened Premenstrual Syndrome (PMS).** Some women are more sensitive to hormonal fluctuations and/ or their hormones are unbalanced leading to premenstrual syndrome (PMS). The symptoms of PMS are exacerbated during perimenopause because hormone fluctuations occur more frequently than just monthly and because perimenopause can lead to significant imbalances in hormones.

Hot Tip: I wish I had known this thirty years ago. Bad PMS over the course of many years is actually a sign our hormones are not in balance. About a third of women experience PMS and as a result, PMS has become somewhat normalized. If you have a child or a friend with bad PMS who is not in perimenopause, encourage them to dig deeper into their hormones as there's a likely culprit. My decades of bad PMS were likely due to an imbalance between estrogen and progesterone that worsened the week prior to my period.

- **Decreased Sex Drive.** Many women begin to lose interest in sex during perimenopause. I cover this topic extensively in Chapter 15.

- **Breast Tenderness.** Sore, swollen breasts are a good sign you are in perimenopause, especially if this symptom is new. I remember the first month my breasts swelled up and felt tender and I wondered if I was pregnant because I hadn't experienced that kind of swelling and pain since early pregnancy.

- **Fatigue.** Many of us are downright exhausted in perimenopause. For some of us, that exhaustion is a result of balancing our families, our careers and other responsibilities. For others of us, the fatigue is due to hot flashes that awaken us in the middle of the night. Still others experience fatigue due to hormone imbalances: often too little testosterone or progesterone. You may be surprised to see testosterone mentioned here as many of us consider testosterone a male hormone. I talk about the importance of testosterone for women in great detail in future chapters, especially Chapters 4, 7, 10 and 15.

- **Brain Fog and Forgetfulness.** Many women in perimenopause experience brain fog or find themselves forgetting things for the first time in their lives due to decreased estrogen. The Department of Health and Human Services' Office of Women's Health says up to two-thirds of women in perimenopause report cognitive problems.[11] This was one of the scariest symptoms for me. I think for a living, and I couldn't seem to do it anymore. My brain felt like it wasn't firing like it was supposed to.

- **Weight Gain.** The reality is that our metabolism slows down as we age. If we don't adjust the amount of food we eat or increase the amount of calories we expend, many of us end up gaining weight. Imbalanced hormones, including the imbalance between estrogen and progesterone, which is more common in perimenopause, can also lead to weight gain. Hypothyroid disease is often diagnosed during perimenopause, which can further affect our metabolism. More information about estrogen dominance can be found in

---

11 Weber, M., Mapstone, M., Staskiewicz, J., Maki, P.M. (2012). Reconciling subjective memory complaints with objective memory performance in the menopausal transition. *Menopause;* 19: 735–741.

Chapter 6 and information on thyroid disease is available in Chapter 5.

• **Migraines and Headaches.** Estimates show that up to 85 percent of perimenopausal women experience tension headaches, and up to 29 percent suffer from migraines.[12] A study that surveyed more than thirty thousand migraine sufferers found that migraine frequency increased 60 percent during perimenopause.[13]

• **Mood Changes.** Approximately 30 percent of women in perimenopause experience mood changes.[14] Can you blame us given all of the hormone shifts some of us experience??! Chapter 13 offers detailed information about the emotional and mental health issues associated with perimenopause.

• **Trouble Sleeping.** About 40 percent of perimenopausal women have sleep problems, including trouble falling

---

12   Ripa, Patrizia et al. "Migraine in menopausal women: A systematic review." *International journal of women's health* vol. 7 773–782. 20 Aug. 2015, doi:10.2147/IJWH.S70073

13   Vincent T. Martin, Jelena Pavlovic, Kristina M. Fanning, Dawn C. Buse, Michael L. Reed, Richard B. Lipton. **Perimenopause and Menopause Are Associated With High Frequency Headache in Women With Migraine: Results of the American Migraine Prevalence and Prevention Study**. *Headache: The Journal of Head and Face Pain*, 2016; DOI: 10.1111/head.12763

14   Bromberger, Joyce T, and Howard M Kravitz. "Mood and menopause: Findings from the Study of Women's Health Across the Nation (SWAN) over 10 years." *Obstetrics and gynecology clinics of North America* vol. 38,3 (2011): 609–625. doi:10.1016/j.ogc.2011.05.011

asleep or inability to stay asleep.[15] For some women this is due to night sweats and for others it's increased anxiety and decreasing melatonin levels.

- **Urinary Urgency, Infection and Leakage.** In perimenopause our estrogen levels decrease, which can result in urogenital atrophy, which is the deterioration of the urinary tract and vagina. A lack of estrogen also reduces the urinary tract's ability to control urination. We may feel the need to urinate more frequently, find ourselves unable to control urination or experience increased urinary tract infections.

- **Vaginal Dryness and Infections.** Due to decreased levels of estrogen, many women experience vaginal dryness during perimenopause, which can cause pain during sex. Vaginal infections may also occur more frequently.

- **Depression.** As many as 30 percent of women in perimenopause experience depression. For women who have a history of depression, that figure can be as high as 59 percent.[16] Depression may be due to fluctuating hormones, stress in midlife and lack of sleep. Women who experience depression in perimenopause may find themselves

15   Joffe H, Massler A, Sharkey KM. Evaluation and management of sleep disturbance during the menopause transition. Semin Reprod Med. 2010 Sep;28(5):404–421. doi: 10.1055/s-0030-1262900. Epub 2010 Sep 15. PMID: 20845239; PMCID: PMC3736837.

16   Bromberger, J., Schott, L., Kravitz, H., & Joffe, H. (2015). Risk factors for major depression during midlife among a community sample of women with and without prior major depression: Are they the same or different? *Psychological Medicine, 45*(8), 1653–1664. doi:10.1017/S0033291714002773

more irritable versus sad or fearful. I discuss the mental and emotional aspects of perimenopause in great detail in Chapter 13.

- **Heart Palpitations.** Anywhere from 18.6 to 46.8 percent of women will experience heart palpitations in later perimenopause and into menopause as estrogen levels decrease quickly.[17] These palpitations are often described as loud, racing or skipped heartbeats, flip-flops, fluttering or pounding that occurs with or without dizziness or light-headedness. Heart palpitations can be very scary, especially if we are not aware that they are a common symptom in both perimenopause and menopause. Unfortunately, there is a lot the medical community still does not know about what causes heart palpitations in midlife. It's important to see a doctor if you experience heart palpitations to ensure you do not have cardiovascular concerns.

- **Hair Changes, Hair loss.** Many women experience changes to their hair in menopause that worsen later in perimenopause and into menopause. These changes include hair looking thinner, hair breakage, hair appearing frizzy and damaged and hair loss. These issues are likely a direct result of decreasing estrogen and progesterone in perimenopause and menopause although stress, extreme dieting, thyroid issues and genetics may also play a part.

---

17 Sievert, Lynnette Leidy, and Carla Makhlouf Obermeyer. "Symptom clusters at midlife: A four-country comparison of checklist and qualitative responses." *Menopause (New York, N.Y.)* vol. 19,2 (2012): 133–144. doi:10.1097/gme.0b013e3182292af3

IMPORTANT NOTE 1: While research on perimenopause is still lacking, the SWAN study, which followed a cohort of Hispanic, Japanese, Chinese, Black and White women in seven cities for more than two decades, found differences in perimenopause and menopause symptoms based on race and ethnicity. For example, the study found Black women have the highest prevalence and longest duration, and are the most bothered by hot flashes, while White women have a lower composite strength in bones. Black and Hispanic women also experience poorer-quality sleep, which could affect cardiovascular health. *Bromberger, Joyce T, and Howard M Kravitz. "Mood and menopause: findings from the Study of Women's Health Across the Nation (SWAN) over 10 years." Obstetrics and gynecology clinics of North America vol. 38,3 (2011): 609–625. doi:10.1016/j. ogc.2011.05.011*

IMPORTANT NOTE 2: It's important to point out that while these are the most common signs of perimenopause, some very fortunate women—approximately one in four or 25 percent— experience *no* perimenopause symptoms at all.

II. Most Common Signs and Symptoms of Menopause

Remember menopause is the time in which you have not had a menstrual period for twelve months. That does not necessarily mean the end of the signs and symptoms of perimenopause. In fact, in menopause we are susceptible to most of the symptoms we may experience in perimenopause due to fluctuating and decreasing hormone levels. The two exceptions are migraines and headaches and worsened PMS. Many women find migraines and headaches disappear in menopause because hormone fluctuations are less frequent. Similarly, if we are not supplementing our hormones in any way, a subject I dive into in the next chapter, we may find that because we are no longer cycling, our PMS symptoms decrease or disappear altogether.

III. Most Common Signs and Symptoms of Postmenopause

The postmenopausal stage is the time after we've no longer had a period for a full year. During this stage, menopausal symptoms such as hot flashes may ease for many of us. However, some women continue to experience menopausal symptoms for a decade or longer after the menopause transition. As a result of a lower level of estrogen, postmenopausal women are at increased risk for a number of health conditions such as osteoporosis and heart disease. I talk about this in greater detail in the next chapter.

My hope is that this chapter has given you an understanding of the stages of women's reproductive health beginning in our thirties and the signs and symptoms to look out for during these stages. When we know what to look for, we can prepare, we can advocate for ourselves and we can take steps that will help us thrive in each of these stages. I highly encourage you to tune into yourself. Familiarize yourself with your body, track any symptoms you may be feeling and share them with your care team. Onward!

FINAL NOTE: PREGNANCY AND PERIMENOPAUSE. It is very important for all women in perimenopause to understand that their chances of becoming pregnant do not decrease in perimenopause. While some of our periods become irregular, if you are having menstrual cycles it means you are still releasing eggs for fertilization and can get pregnant. In the 1950s, 1960s and 1970s there was a phrase: "change of life babies." These children were conceived during perimenopause when women's cycles had become irregular. Some women believed they were going through "the change," which is what menopause was euphemistically called at the time, and believed they couldn't become pregnant, so they stopped using birth control. And then, bam! A new baby at age forty-three. I know many women who are trying to conceive in their forties. This is good news for them! However, for those of you who do not wish to become pregnant in perimenopause, please use birth control.

Chapter 4:

_____

HORMONES ARE EVERYTHING!

> **"I'VE LOST THE ABILITY TO SLEEP THROUGH**
> the night. I'm so exhausted by the end of the day that I fall asleep
> immediately, but I wake up every morning at three thirty or four
> thirty and can't fall back to sleep. I lie there frustrated, filled with
> anxiety and sometimes sweating from a hot flash. I wish I knew
> what was happening to me. It's nearly impossible for me to get
> through each day without bursting into tears. I'm not sure if it's
> exhaustion or hormones." —*Tamika*

In this chapter I'm going to get a little "science-y" (but not too much!)
and dive deep into hormones. Before perimenopause I hadn't thought
much about hormones since I was a teenager when my body suddenly
took on a life of its own due to a sudden influx of hormones. The reality is that our bodies at middle age are going through a very similar
phenomenon as they did when we were teenagers, only instead of an
influx of hormones, we experience the slow and steady departure of
hormones. To thrive in perimenopause we need to know:

- Why hormones are important.

- What they do.

- What happens to our hormones in perimenopause.

- Why balanced hormones are key to feeling well.

Let's dive in!

WHAT ARE HORMONES?

Hormones are chemical substances that act like messenger molecules in the body. After being made in one part of the body, they travel to other parts of the body where they help control how cells and organs do their work. In this chapter I go into detail on five specific hormones:

MAJOR SEX HORMONES

Estrogen

Estrogen is made by both men and women, but it is more predominant in women. It is a serious workhorse with impact on both gender and reproduction, but on much else as well.

Where Does Estrogen Come From?

The ovaries, which produce a woman's eggs, are the main source of estrogen in your body. Your adrenal glands, located at the top of each kidney, also make small amounts of estrogen, as does fat tissue.

What Does Estrogen Do?

In puberty estrogen is responsible for the growth of the breasts, the growth of pubic and underarm hair and the start of menstrual cycles. After puberty estrogen controls our menstrual cycles and is key to childbearing. It keeps cholesterol in control, protects our bones, affects our brains (including mood) and plays a big part in a range of organs, vessels and tissues. Estrogen moves through your blood and acts everywhere in your body.

WHAT HAPPENS TO ESTROGEN LEVELS IN PERIMENOPAUSE AND HOW DO THEY AFFECT US?

In our menstrual years estrogen levels change throughout the month. They are highest in the middle of our menstrual cycle and lowest during our period. Our estrogen levels decrease as we age and they fluctuate in perimenopause. Those changes in levels cause the signs and symptoms of perimenopause I discussed in the previous chapter, including:

- Menstrual periods that are less frequent or stop.

- Hot flashes and/or night sweats.

- Trouble sleeping.

- Dryness and thinning of the vagina.

- Low sexual desire.

- Brain fog.

- Mood swings.

- Dry skin.

- Migraines and headaches.

Some women have such high levels of estrogen compared to other hormones that it causes an imbalance, possibly starting prior to perimenopause and continuing into perimenopause. This can occur for many reasons, including the use of birth control pills. I happen to be one of these women. In other words, despite the fact that my estrogen level is decreasing as I age, it's still outsized compared to my progesterone and testosterone levels. This is known as estrogen dominance. You can learn more about estrogen dominance in Chapter 6.

Progesterone

Progesterone is the hormone that plays a large role in our fertility and menstruation and is essential to the survival of a fetus.

Where Does Progesterone Come From?

Progesterone is made primarily in our ovaries, although a small amount is also produced in our adrenal glands. Most of our progesterone is made in the second half of our menstrual cycles. It is secreted by the corpus luteum, a temporary endocrine gland the female body produces after ovulation.

What Does Progesterone Do?

Progesterone doesn't have quite the "dynamo" reputation that estrogen does, but it's no less of a powerhouse. Progesterone is the hormone that controls our well-being. It helps us feel calm and it raises our body temperature, which in turn helps our metabolism. Progesterone is mother nature's diuretic, helping us get rid of excess body fluids. Progesterone is the soothing hormone, which is why when our progesterone levels lower just prior to our periods, so many of us experience PMS. That's because: "Progesterone has left the building!"

From a more technical perspective, progesterone prepares the endometrium (the lining of the uterus) for the potential of pregnancy after ovulation. It tells the lining to thicken to accept a fertilized egg. It also makes sure our uterus doesn't contract and reject any fertilized eggs. When our bodies are told to create high levels of progesterone, we will not ovulate. If, on the other hand, an egg is not fertilized, the corpus luteum breaks down, lowering the progesterone levels in the body, and we begin to menstruate.

What Happens to Progesterone Levels in Perimenopause and How Do They Affect Us?

Similar to estrogen levels, progesterone levels fluctuate month to month and year to year. The most important thing to remember with progesterone is that progesterone is the "yin" to estrogen's "yang." The goal is to have the appropriate amounts of each and to have those levels shift back and forth seamlessly, maintaining a balance between the two. Unfortunately, that balance can be challenging for many of us and worsens in perimenopause because in perimenopause we begin to have menstrual cycles in which we don't release eggs for fertilization. These non-egg-releasing cycles result in a rise in estrogen levels and a sharp decline in progesterone. Without the balancing effect of progesterone, estrogen begins to get out of control, resulting in some of the signs and symptoms of perimenopause I discussed in the previous chapter, including:

- Migraines.

- Irritability.

- Rage.

- Heavy periods.

- Unpredictable cycles.

- Painful, swollen breasts.

- Weepiness.

- Water retention.

- Weight gain.

- Decreased sex drive.

Testosterone

Based on my conversations with women, testosterone is the hormone few women know a lot about. Yet the reality is that testosterone is just as important to women's health as estrogen and progesterone! Testosterone is part of a group of hormones known as androgens, which in larger quantities produce male traits and reproductive characteristics, such as the development of the penis and the testes.

Where Does Testosterone Come From?

Testosterone is produced in women's ovaries as well as the adrenal glands.

What Does Testosterone Do?

While testosterone might fly under the radar for a lot of us, it has very important functions, including:

- Contributing to our libido.

- Playing a role in our estrogen production.

- Helping maintain bone mass.

- Building muscle.

- Helping with muscle recovery and body pain.

What Happens to Testosterone Levels in Perimenopause and How Do They Affect Us?

Women's testosterone levels are at their highest when we're in our twenties and then decline slowly from that point on. Some women produce too much testosterone in their twenties, and that often results in irregular or absent menstrual periods, more body hair and acne. By the time we're in our forties our testosterone levels are at half of their peak. This means that for many of us perimenopause is a time in which we experience:

- Decreased sexual desire.

- Decreased sexual satisfaction.

- Depressed mood.

- Decreased energy.

- Muscle weakness and pain.

- Vaginal dryness.

MY TESTOSTERONE STORY: According to the Boston University School of Medicine, a fifty-year-old woman's total testosterone level is considered low if it's less than 25 ng/dL. Testosterone levels lower than 20 ng/dL in women aged fifty and older are considered very low. When my testosterone levels were tested shortly after I turned forty-eight they were 11 ng/dL. SO LOW! No wonder I was exhausted all the time. My body was turning to Jell-O and my sex drive was under attack!

Testosterone is very important to our health and well-being. Low testosterone levels in women may occur due to:[18]

- Adrenal insufficiency.

- Hypopituitarism, which is when your pituitary gland doesn't release adequate levels of hormones.

- Oral estrogen therapy, including the combined oral contraceptive pill.

- Oophorectomy—surgical removal of the ovaries.

- Chemical oophorectomy—ovarian failure caused by certain medication, such as gonadotropin-releasing hormone antagonists, chemotherapy or radiotherapy.

- Hyperprolactinaemia—overproduction of the pituitary hormone prolactin.

- Premature ovarian failure—early menopause (before the age of forty), with various causes.

Keep in mind that adrenal insufficiency and hypopituitarism are linked to thyroid disease, so check out Chapter 5 for more information.

ADDITIONAL HORMONES

While estrogen, progesterone and testosterone are major sex hormones, many more hormones are circulating in your body. I go

---

18 Gleicher, N., Kushnir, V.A., Weghofer, A. *et al.* The importance of adrenal hypoandrogenism in infertile women with low functional ovarian reserve: A case study of associated adrenal insufficiency. *Reprod Biol Endocrinol* 14, 23 (2016). https://doi.org/10.1186/s12958-016-0158-9

into detail here about four additional hormones because they each often play a role in perimenopause.

Adrenal Hormones

Our adrenal glands are small, triangular-shaped glands located on top of both of our kidneys. They secrete cortisol and aldosterone and are responsible for regulating our metabolism, immune system, blood pressure and response to stress. Our adrenal glands also control mineral balance, produce adrenaline and control our blood sugar levels. When our adrenal glands don't produce enough cortisol and aldosterone this can lead to Addison's disease.

The adrenal glands also produce steroid hormones such as DHEA and some estrogen, progesterone and testosterone. However, when we are under pressure, the adrenals prioritize the production of adrenaline and cortisol instead of the sex hormones. This means constant stress can affect the availability of key sex hormones. Many of us are in "go, go, go" mode 24/7. Stress has become a way of life for us. When we are living in "fight, flight or freeze" mode most of the time our adrenals become overworked. They are dealing with the constant production of adrenalin, which increases our heart rate and raises our blood sugar levels to give us the energy our body thinks it needs to respond to whatever threat is causing us stress. Ultimately, this constant use of adrenal hormones can lead to what some people call "adrenal fatigue," which isn't actually a medical diagnosis and is considered controversial in the medical community. I don't think it's worthwhile to argue whether adrenal fatigue exists. What I do want to underscore is that overtaxing our adrenals is not a good thing and can affect the availability of our sex hormones, so it's important to address stress in our lives. More on that in Chapters 11 and 13!

DHEA

Dehydroepiandrosterone (DHEA) is a natural steroid our bodies naturally produce in our adrenal glands. DHEA helps produce other hormones, including estrogen, progesterone and testosterone. Our DHEA levels peak in early adulthood and then slowly decrease as we age. Women's DHEA levels decrease more quickly than men's levels. The most dramatic fall in DHEA occurs between the ages of twenty and thirty and then again between the ages of forty and fifty, when levels drop by 60–70 percent. Because DHEA is a precursor to the sex hormones, when DHEA levels falls they lead to decreases in those sex hormones, which leads to the symptoms I discussed in the previous chapter, including dry skin and thinning of the vaginal wall. When we overtax our adrenals it makes it harder to produce DHEA.

Thyroid

Our thyroids are a powerhouse hormone and many women experience thyroid issues during perimenopause. For that reason, I dedicate the entire next chapter (5) to this topic. Go there for in-depth information on the thyroid hormone.

Cortisol

Cortisol is our body's main stress hormone. It controls our mood, motivation and fear. Cortisol is made by our adrenal glands and plays an important role in many of our bodily functions, including:

- Managing how our body uses carbohydrates, fats and proteins.

- Managing inflammation.

- Managing energy.

- Regulating blood pressure and increasing blood sugar.

- Controlling sleep and wake cycles.

As we go into perimenopause and we are producing smaller amounts of progesterone, which is the feel-good, calming hormone, we have less of a buffer against stress. Without that buffer we feel stress (and we likely have more of it at this time of life!) all the more, so our bodies will respond to it more. Our bodies produce two hormones in our adrenal glands when we are under stress: cortisol and adrenaline. Cortisol can also reduce our ability to produce progesterone, so we find ourselves in an even more extreme low-progesterone/high-cortisol loop. High cortisol levels can result in the following symptoms:

- Insomnia.

- Low energy, even if getting adequate sleep.

- Frequent colds.

- Cravings for unhealthy foods.

- Digestion problems like bloating.

- Weight gain, especially around the middle.

- Low sex drive.

- More aches and pains.

- Low mood.

THE HORMONE DANCE OR ORCHESTRA

At this point in this chapter, you may be wondering why I've spent so much time going into the details of each specific hormone. I did so intentionally because maintaining a balance between these hormones is key to our overall well-being. Keep in mind that while I only went into detail about seven hormones, our endocrine system actually has one hundred hormones circulating the body. One hundred! That's a lot of hormones to keep in balance.

I like to think of each of our hormones as working together in a choreographed dance with specific steps. You could also think of these hormones as an orchestra, with each instrument or hormone responsible for a certain role, while at the same time also being responsible for its interactions with the other instruments or hormones within the orchestra.

The challenge in achieving hormone balance is that our hormone levels are unique to each of us and the signs and symptoms we experience in perimenopause are directly related to those levels. In other words, while my testosterone levels tanked first in perimenopause, my best friend's estrogen levels were the first thing to go. How do you know which of your hormones are in balance and which are not? A good care team will ask you what you're feeling and what changes to your physical, emotional and mental health you're noticing, if any. They will also test your hormones regularly. You can also test your own hormones. I have not done this myself, but check out these companies as a starting point: **Everlywell, Modern Fertility, LetsGetChecked** and **myLab Box.**

The other challenge with balancing hormones is that there are many ways in which our hormones can become imbalanced. Hormone imbalances come from our body making too much or too little of a hormone or several hormones. Perimenopause is one reason our hormones may be out of imbalance. An illness like diabetes may be another reason our hormones are out of balance. Injury, toxins, trauma, sleep issues and stress may also cause hormonal imbalances. In fact, sleep issues and stress are two huge culprits when it comes to hormonal imbalances, which is why I dedicate Chapters 11, 12 and 13 to those very topics. My hope is that knowing what each hormone is expected to do and what may happen in perimenopause will help you be prepared when speaking with your health-care team. You've got this!

Note: Some content in this chapter also comes from:

www.aarp.org/health/conditions-treatments/info-2018/menopause-symptoms-doctors-relief-treatment.html

www.hormone.org/your-health-and-hormones/glands-and-hormones-a-to-z/hormones/progesterone

Chapter 5:

DON'T IGNORE YOUR THYROID

"I WENT TO DOCTOR AFTER DOCTOR AND they all told me my labs looked fine. They refused to treat me. My hair was falling out and I was so depressed I couldn't get out of bed most days. My whole body hurt, and I had gained twenty-five pounds. How could anyone think I was fine? Most of the doctors urged me to try antidepressants, but I was already on them and they weren't working. I knew there was something wrong with me physically. I still don't understand why no one listened to me." — *Lauren*

At the risk of putting you to sleep with too many statistics, I need to drop some numbers here:[19]

- An estimated *20 million Americans* have some form of thyroid disease. The majority of them are unaware of their condition.

---

19 This chapter is highly influenced by the 2019 hard-copy book *Stop the Thyroid Madness: A Patient Revolution against Decades of Inferior Thyroid Treatment* (STTM) written by Janie A. Bowthorpe, as well as my own thyroid experience. All statistics in this chapter come from STTM.

- Not only that, but women are *five to eight times* more likely than men to have thyroid problems.

- In fact, *one in eight women* will develop a thyroid disorder during her lifetime. An underactive thyroid affects women up to fifteen times more often than men.

I don't know about you, but with these kinds of statistics, I would argue that thyroid disease is an epidemic among women in the United States. But, because there is very little awareness about thyroid disease, it's a hidden epidemic.

During my perimenopause journey, I experienced symptoms for many, many frustrating years. I now know some of those symptoms were directly related to thyroid disease. At the time I shared with my health-care team the following symptoms:

- I was hungry all the time.

- I had intense cravings for salt.

- I was gaining weight despite eating well and exercising.

- I felt intense fatigue at all times.

- I was feeling depressed despite being on antidepressants.

- I always felt cold, wearing thick socks even in 95 degree weather.

Despite voicing my concerns repeatedly, I was told my thyroid levels were normal and my symptoms didn't warrant treatment. What I didn't know at the time is that for many women, their thyroid journey resembles the experience of women in perimenopause. After reading many books on thyroid disease and reading hundreds of women's thyroid stories I noticed some trends:

- There is not enough research done on thyroid disease.

- Clinicians use outdated testing methods to diagnose thyroid disease.

- Clinicians prescribe treatments that at best do nothing and at worst lead to additional health problems.

- Women's needs are unmet and their concerns are ignored or belittled.

Here's the kicker. The risk of thyroid disease increases in perimenopause.

Just like perimenopause, you need to know the symptoms of thyroid disease to prepare yourself. If you have thyroid disease symptoms, it is highly likely you will need to advocate for yourself and for effective treatment. Let's dive in!

WHAT IS THE THYROID AND WHAT DOES IT DO?

The thyroid gland is a small organ located in the front of the neck, wrapped around the windpipe. It's shaped like a butterfly, smaller in the middle with two wide wings that extend around the side of your throat. It's incredible how many aspects of our physical and mental health and well-being are affected by the thyroid! Your thyroid affects every system in your body and if it's not functioning properly, you will not either.

Your thyroid has one particularly important job to do within your body. It releases and controls hormones that are in charge of your metabolism and affect blood pressure, breathing, digestion, energy levels, body temperature and nerve function. Your thyroid controls your metabolism via hormones. Your metabolism is like a generator.

It takes in raw energy and uses it to power your body. Metabolism is the process where the food you eat is transformed into energy. This energy is used throughout your entire body to keep many of your body's systems working correctly. Your metabolism is made up of two hormones—T4 or thyroxine and T3 or triiodothyronine. T3 and T4 hormones are created by the thyroid and they tell your cells how much energy to use. When your thyroid works correctly, it maintains the appropriate amount of hormones to keep your metabolism working at the right rate.

The inner workings of your metabolism and thyroid are supervised by your pituitary gland, which is in the center of the skull below your brain. The pituitary gland monitors and controls the amount of thyroid hormones in your bloodstream. When the pituitary gland senses a lack of thyroid hormones or a high level of hormones in your body, it will adjust the amounts with its own hormone. This hormone is called thyroid-stimulating hormone (TSH). The TSH will be sent to the thyroid and it will tell the thyroid what needs to be done to get the body back to normal.

When problems occur with your thyroid it means the pituitary gland makes too little or too much thyroid hormone and this affects a myriad of things. You likely have a thyroid issue if you have:

- Unexplained weight gain or loss.

- Joint pain.

- Wired and agitated nervous system.

- Loss of sex drive.

- Fibrocystic breasts.

- Hair loss, brittle hair.

- Dry skin.

- Dry eyes.

- Slightly bulging eyeballs.

TYPES OF THYROID DISEASE

Let's dig in some more to the specific types of thyroid disease:

Hyperthyroidism (Grave's Disease)

If your body makes too much thyroid hormone, you may develop hyperthyroidism, which can make your metabolism speed up. Symptoms of hyperthyroidism include a rapid heartbeat, weight loss, increased appetite and anxiety.

Hypothyroidism

If your body makes too little thyroid hormone, it's called hypothyroidism. When you don't have enough thyroid hormone in your body, you feel tired, you might gain weight and you may have a low body temperature, making you feel cold at all times. Hypothyroidism is much more common than hyperthyroidism and it typically occurs after age forty, around the same time as perimenopause.

Hashimoto's Thyroiditis

Hashimoto's is less common than both hyperthyroidism and hypothyroidism. It occurs when the body's immune system produces antibodies that destroy the thyroid over time, preventing the thyroid gland from making enough thyroid hormone. Symptoms of Hashimoto's include enlarged thyroid or neck goiter, which can make swallowing difficult, unexplained weight gain, fatigue, puffiness in the face, depression and inability to get warm.

The Perimenopause–Thyroid Connection

When we are entering perimenopause, it's important to be on the look-out for issues with our thyroid. That's because women go through per-imenopause in midlife and the likelihood of hypothyroidism increases as we age, especially for women. For lucky (haha!) women like me, perimenopause and the diagnosis of hypothyroidism may happen at the same time. It took a while for my clinicians to realize I was strug-gling with both perimenopause and thyroid disease, probably because so many of the symptoms overlap. Thyroid disease requires its own treatment, so it is important to get an accurate assessment.

Not only do the symptoms of thyroid disease and perimeno-pause overlap but thyroid hormones and estrogen hormones can influence each other and exacerbate symptoms. To make matters more confusing, sometimes hypothyroidism and perimenopause are mistaken for one another because they are both associated with weight gain and increased fatigue. The thyroid gland keeps our metabolism in balance so with too little thyroid hormones our metabolism runs more slowly and we can't burn off calories efficiently.

Many perimenopausal women also gain weight because of estro-gen levels that are higher than normal and progesterone levels that are too low. Additionally, higher estrogen levels or estrogen dominance can cause weight gain because of insulin resistance (more on estrogen dominance in Chapter 6). Insulin resistance is when cells in our mus-cles, fat and liver don't respond well to insulin and can't use glucose from our blood for energy. Over time, our blood sugar levels go up and we store fat, frequently in our abdominals.

The ups and downs in estrogen that occur during perimeno-pause also directly influence thyroid function because estrogen reg-ulates the hormone-binding protein called thyroid-binding globulin

(TBG). When estrogen levels are high, the liver produces more TBG, dropping the thyroid's output of T3 and T4. This leads to the symptoms listed earlier until the thyroid gland is stimulated to produce more. When estrogen levels temporarily drop, during a skipped menstrual cycle of perimenopause, for example, TBG levels also drop so the amount of "free" T3 and T4 increases temporarily, leading to a hyperthyroid imbalance. Again, for some women, weight gain and fatigue may be an indication of perimenopause or it may mean a thyroid issue. That's where diagnosis comes in and I wish I could say it was an easy path, but for many, including me, it's anything but easy!

Diagnosing Thyroid Disease

I've been studying thyroid disease and treatment since I was diagnosed, and I'm very concerned about the way thyroid disease is diagnosed in the United States.[20] I cannot stress this enough: it is extremely important for you to know what to ask for when it comes to diagnosis, or you will remain untreated and over time will experience significant health challenges.

Most clinicians rely on blood tests *alone* to diagnose thyroid disease.[21] This is a MAJOR PROBLEM! Blood tests may appear "normal" despite common thyroid symptoms. This is because many clinicians use outdated levels and optimal ranges to diagnose hypothyroid. Not only that, but thyroid hormone levels should not be the only indicator of whether a patient does or does not have thyroid disease. Thousands of patients are told every year (I was one of them) that their thyroid

---

20   I learned a tremendous amount about thyroid diagnoses after spending years in private online thyroid groups talking to and listening to women about their personal experiences.

21   Bowthorpe, Janie A. *Stop the Thyroid Madness: A Patient Revolution Against Decades of Inferior Thyroid Treatment*, 2019.

levels are healthy, despite the fact that they feel awful, and learned later that they did indeed have thyroid disease. Here's what you need to know:

Don't Fall for the Thyroid-Stimulating Hormone Myth. The TSH test is one of the most commonly prescribed thyroid lab tests worldwide. It is believed to be a reliable way to assess thyroid function. However, hundreds of thousands of people who are suffering from thyroid disease symptoms get TSH test results in the "normal" range. Using TSH to assess thyroid is not supported by the vast majority of functional and integrative clinicians. Many traditional clinicians have also begun to realize testing TSH is not a useful way to assess thyroid function, but many others refuse to budge.

Hot Tip: If you are experiencing any of the symptoms I've listed, ask your health-care team to test your total T3 and T4 levels. If they insist on testing TSH instead, find a new care team and/or test the levels yourself using a home kit from a company like **LetsGetChecked.**

Test your FREE T3 and T4 levels. In addition to testing your total T3 and 4 levels, it is important to test your *free* T3 and T4 levels. Free T3 and T4 are the levels of these hormones that are free, available and usable in your blood serum. It's important to insist on testing free T3 and T4 because when you test the total hormone you don't have any idea how much of that hormone is actually available and usable.

TREATING THYROID DISEASE

Here's where things get very frustrating. Not only can it be difficult to get an accurate thyroid diagnosis, getting appropriate treatment can be an absolute nightmare. Here are three of the most common things to be aware of:

T4 Treatment Alone Will Not Help Hypothyroid Thyroid.[22]

An epidemic of poor hypothyroid treatment is occurring in the United States and a lot of it has to do with a reliance on T4 medication only. This T4 medicine is known as levothyroxine sodium, also called l-thyroxine or T4. Brand names of this medicine include Synthroid, Tirosint, Levothroid, Elyroxin, Oroxine and Unithroid. There's also generic Levothyroxine.

Patients on T4 treatment alone may feel slightly better initially but ultimately none of their thyroid symptoms are managed. I have spoken with many women who are depressed, overweight and exhausted with brain fog. They believe the T4 medication they're taking is managing their hypothyroidism and yet they are suffering daily from common hypothyroid symptoms. How can this be? The problem with T4-only treatment is that T4 is a *storage* hormone that is ineffective on its own in doing all the things the thyroid gland is supposed to do. T4 must be converted to T3, which is the active hormone. Our bodies require this active hormone to work at certain levels for the thyroid to fully do its job. If you have been diagnosed with hypothyroid disease, it is *very important* you are treated with both T4 and T3 medication. This is nonnegotiable because T3 levels are responsible for creating your body's energy and affect your overall health and well-being. If your health-care team refuses to treat you with both T3 and T4, please *run* and find a new care team or you risk joining the millions of women in this country whose thyroid disease is not managed appropriately.

---

22   Bowthorpe, *Stop the Thyroid Madness.*

Do Not Fall For the Titration Method or Low Levels of Medication.

T4-only treatment is not the only reason millions of women suffer with hypothyroid symptoms despite taking medicine every day. The other reason so many of us don't feel better after starting thyroid medicine is because our health-care team either puts us on a low dose and keeps us there or titrates us up very, very slowly, resulting in continued hypothyroid symptoms. I've read hundreds of women's stories. They are all similar and they all mirror my own.

I was so relieved when I was finally diagnosed with thyroid disease and was told I would start taking T3 and T4. I was desperate to feel better and had high hopes the medication would get me there. Unfortunately, the dose I was put on was so low it improved my symptoms only slightly. I repeatedly spoke with my health-care team sharing the list of symptoms I continued to deal with on a daily basis. They slowly, and I mean very slowly, raised my dosage. It was excruciating to wait weeks and weeks to feel better. Ultimately I hit a dose that alleviated *every single one* of my symptoms. Here's the thing I have realized after talking with and learning from many, many thyroid patients: most of us require higher thyroid medicine doses than what is traditionally believed to be acceptable.

If the experiences of millions of women with hypothyroid disease are any indication, you will need to advocate for yourself. For many of us, low dosages of T4 and T3 will not adequately replace the thyroid hormone our bodies are missing. If your health-care team insists on starting you at a low dose, you must request an increase of medicine every couple of days until your symptoms have disappeared. If your health-care team refuses to increase your dose, find a new health-care team. If they use TSH levels as an excuse for not increasing your dose, know that it is perfectly normal for you to go below range.

Not only that, reread the section above about the TSH myth. TSH tests are not an effective way to assess thyroid functioning!

Make Sure You Check Your Cortisol and Iron Levels

I stand by everything I just shared regarding thyroid medicine dosages; however, you may run into problems when raising thyroid medicine doses if your cortisol levels are not healthy or you have inadequate iron levels. If our cortisol levels are not right, thyroid medicine can give us hyper symptoms: we feel shaky and anxious, we have trouble sleeping or we can continue to feel hypothyroid. The same issue occurs with inadequate levels of iron. I highly recommend testing both iron and cortisol if you suspect you may be hypothyroid and address any issues prior to beginning medication treatment.

Be Aware of Desiccated Thyroid Issues (Beginning in 2014)

As if everything with thyroid disease wasn't already complicated, the last issue I want to be sure you're aware of is desiccated thyroid medicine. If you have been diagnosed with hypothyroid disease, you may have heard of desiccated thyroid. Brands of desiccated thyroid medication include Armour, Nature Thyroid, NP Thyroid and WP Thyroid. In the United States, desiccated thyroid medicine is almost exclusively made up of the thyroid glands of pigs. In some countries like New Zealand and Argentina, desiccated thyroid medicine is made of the thyroid from grass-fed cows.

Desiccated thyroid medicine has been used to treat thyroid disease since the late 1800s, and many patients like it because it's natural and it contains both T3 and T4, which gives you the exact two hormones you're missing if you have hypothyroid disease. I was a huge fan of desiccated thyroid medicine when I was first diagnosed because it made my hypothyroid symptoms disappear—at first.

Here's the problem: since 2014, patients in the United States have expressed concern that desiccated thyroid medicine isn't working for them like it once did, and their lab results are confirming those concerns. Patient concerns were followed by a series of recalls of desiccated thyroid medicines by the US Food and Drug Administration (FDA). For example, in 2020 RLC Labs, Inc. recalled a total of 483 lots of Nature-Thyroid® and WP Thyroid® in all strengths because they were subpotent.[23] In other words, hypothyroid patients weren't getting the doses they needed to address their symptoms. In May 2021 Acella Pharmeuticals voluntarily recalled certain lots of NP Thyroid, its third recall that year.[24]

Fortunately, many other options are available to treat your hypothyroid disease, including medicine from compounding pharmacies and synthetics. I prefer natural treatments whenever possible, but the most important thing is to treat my thyroid symptoms. If the natural versions are not effective, then I am grateful for other options. The most important takeaways I can share with you about thyroid disease and perimenopause are:

- Be aware of thyroid disease symptoms as many women experience thyroid disease during perimenopause.

- Be vigilant about monitoring your symptoms.

- Speak to your doctor if you begin to feel any kinds of hyperthyroid symptoms while on thyroid medication. Your medication may need adjusting.

---

23 www.fda.gov/safety/recalls-market-withdrawals-safety-alerts/rlc-labs-inc-issues-voluntary-nationwide-recall-all-lots-nature-throidr-and-wp-thyroidr-current

24 www.fda.gov/safety/recalls-market-withdrawals-safety-alerts/acella-pharmaceuticals-llc-issues-voluntary-nationwide-recall-certain-lots-np-thyroidr-thyroid-0

- Be your own advocate.

- Work with a care team who tests T3 and T4 levels.

- Work with a care team who treats hypothyroid disease with both T3 and T4 medications.

- Don't rely on TSH tests or stay with a care team who relies exclusively on TSH tests.

- Get labs done regularly to test your thyroid levels.

Chapter 6:

THE NIGHTMARE THAT IS ESTROGEN DOMINANCE

> **"I'VE BEEN AN ATHLETE MY ENTIRE LIFE BUT**
> in my early forties I began to gain weight in my midsection and
> hips. I couldn't gain muscle to save my life. It was like my body
> decided it wanted to hold onto fat for dear life." — *Fatima*

When I was doing the research for this guide I toggled back and forth about whether to include a stand-alone chapter on estrogen dominance. I've struggled with estrogen dominance so I was leaning in that direction, but I didn't want the guide to be biased by my own experiences. What about women who don't have enough estrogen?

Ultimately the numbers and the potential consequences of estrogen dominance are what made me create a stand-alone chapter. The reality is that in perimenopause it's far more likely that you will have too much estrogen than that you will not have enough. That's because while our estrogen levels shift in perimenopause more than ever before, they don't drop significantly until just before, and then again in menopause. In worst-case scenarios, too much estrogen can lead to serious diseases. So let's look at estrogen dominance closely: what it is, why it occurs, the symptoms we experience and the steps we can take to decrease our estrogen levels if we need to.

I hope those of you who do not have estrogen dominance will still learn some interesting strategies that help you in your perimenopause journey. If you do not feel this chapter is relevant to you, please feel free to turn to the next chapter.

What Is Estrogen Dominance?

The main thing to understand about estrogen is that it's metabolized by our liver. If we aren't metabolizing our estrogen efficiently, we may experience estrogen dominance. Some women are estrogen dominant for ten to fifteen years, beginning as early as age thirty-five. There are two ways in which estrogen dominance occurs:

- **Relative estrogen dominance.** You have too much estrogen relative to progesterone

- **Frank estrogen dominance.** Your body simply makes too much estrogen

The term "estrogen dominance" is sometimes used interchangeably with "high estrogen." That doesn't tell the whole story because high estrogen won't make you feel bad if you have enough progesterone to balance it out.

Why Does Estrogen Dominance Happen?

The primary reasons estrogen dominance occurs are:

- An overproduction of estrogen.

- The body does not break down estrogen effectively.

- The body does not excrete estrogen effectively.

Why Is Estrogen Dominance a Problem?

Too much estrogen in our blood can build up and lead to autoimmune disease or to breast cancer, ovarian cancer and other cancer diagnoses. Estrogen dominance can also lead to decreased amounts of available thyroid hormone, which can result in hypothyroid disease, which I wrote about in great detail in Chapter 5.

Hot Tip: As I reflect on my perimenopause journey, I can't help but think that my progesterone levels decreased as I grew older, ultimately making me estrogen dominant in my late thirties, early forties. Over time, thyroid hormone was less available to me due to the estrogen dominance, and ultimately that led to me being diagnosed with hypothyroid disease in my mid-forties. If I had even known estrogen dominance was a "thing" I could have worked with my care team to supplement with progesterone and could have also focused on improving the way my body broke down and excreted estrogen to help it do so effectively. Be on the lookout for any signs of estrogen dominance or low progesterone! They are red flags.

What Causes Estrogen Dominance?

When our menstrual cycle is normal, estrogen is the dominant hormone for the first two weeks leading up to ovulation. In the last two weeks of our cycles, estrogen is balanced by progesterone. As we enter perimenopause we begin to experience anovulatory cycles (which means cycles where no ovulation occurs), making estrogen unopposed and therefore dominant. Skipping ovulation is just one reason we may become estrogen dominant, though a regular and reliable one that most ovulating women experience in perimenopause. Others include:

- Toxins in our environment.

- Too much stress, which results in excess cortisol, insulin and norepinephrine.

- Excess body fat greater than 28 percent.

- A diet with too many bad carbohydrates and not enough fiber, nutrients or high-quality fats.

- Immune issues (e.g., polycystic ovary syndrome [PCOS] or inflammation)

- Poor digestion.

- Poor liver detoxification.

What Are the Symptoms of Estrogen Dominance?

Many of the symptoms of estrogen dominance are similar to the symptoms of perimenopause, likely because estrogen dominance often occurs during perimenopause. With that said, you can experience estrogen dominance before perimenopause. Estrogen dominance symptoms include:

- Irregular periods.

- Bloating.

- Breast swelling and tenderness.

- Fibrocystic breasts.

- Headaches when premenstrual.

- Mood swings.

- Weight and/or fat gain (particularly around the abdomen and hips).

- Hair loss.

- Sluggish metabolism.

- Foggy thinking, memory loss.

- Fatigue.

- Trouble sleeping/insomnia.

- Increased or worsened PMS.

These symptoms may seem familiar because you saw many of them in an earlier chapter when I described the symptoms associated with low progesterone. In a sense, since it always comes down to balance, estrogen dominance can be the same thing as low progesterone.

One of the most frustrating symptoms of estrogen dominance I experienced was increased cellulite. Cellulite is lumpy, dimpled flesh that is actually a harmless skin condition, but for some reason many women feel like it is a personal failing. I admit I was one of those women in late perimenopause. I was eating well, I was exercising, but the cellulite kept showing up. You may know that women tend to have cellulite more than men. That's because the bands of connective tissue under our skin are thinner whereas in men the bands of tissue are thicker, so any fat under our skin shows more easily. Women also tend to have a higher percentage of body fat than men. However, an increase in cellulite in perimenopause has just as much to do with hormone imbalances as it does with skin elasticity and muscle-to-fat ratio. Who knew?! I certainly didn't and I beat myself up the year I turned forty-eight as my body seemed to acquire more cellulite on a daily basis. Looking back, I have a lot of empathy for myself at that time because I was beating myself up for a hormone imbalance, one I didn't even know I had. If you find cellulite cropping up:

- Don't eat less and exercise more!

- Don't feel guilty!

Instead, balance your hormones.

What Can We Do about Estrogen Dominance?

The first step I suggest when it comes to estrogen dominance, and frankly with perimenopause as a whole, is test your hormones! I cannot emphasize enough the importance of testing your hormones regularly in perimenopause. I talk about that in great detail in the next chapter, but the bottom line is that we cannot treat our symptoms unless we know what is causing our symptoms. Furthermore, managing our symptoms comes down to getting our hormones in balance with each other. With all of that said, there are some additional things I recommend when it comes to estrogen dominance:

1. **Clean up your skin care products.** Look closely at your makeup, soap, shampoo, creams and anything else that touches your skin. According to the Environmental Working Group, the average woman uses more than ten different personal care products. The ingredients in those products are easily absorbed through our skin and can find their way into our bloodstream. Avoid any products with the following ingredients:

- Parabens.

- Sodium lauryl or laureth sulfate.

- Fragrance.

- Triclosan.

- Formaldehyde.

- PEGs.

- BHA and BHT.

- Ethanalomines.

- Dibutyl phthalate and toluene.

- Coal tar dyes.

- Hydroquinone.

- Oxybenzone.

You can also go to the Environmental Working Group website at www. ewg.org/ewgverified/index.php to search for any products you have or may be thinking about buying to learn about their toxin levels. I will say this in full transparency: I have not completely overhauled all of the products I use because (a) it's costly to toss out these products and replace them and (2) it's time-consuming. However, I'm slowly but surely moving to products that are less toxic and I will get there eventually.

2. **Help out your liver.** I do whatever I can to help my liver be as effective as possible because the liver is one of the ways estrogen is metabolized. For example, I am fortunate that I can use a sauna regularly and get lymphatic drainage massages every couple of months. I also use a sauna blanket (I use one from

Higher Dose) daily in the winter and multiple times a week the rest of the year. When the liver is forced to work doubly hard to get rid of alcohol, caffeine or environmental toxins its capacity to cleanse the blood of estrogen decreases. Taking a **Milk Thistle** supplement is another way to assist the liver in excreting excess estrogen. I use the **Nature's Bounty** brand.

3. **Find ways to manage stress.** I know this is easier said than done. I get it. I run two companies and I'm on the go all the time, but I've seen firsthand the ways in which stress tears apart my body. The problem with stress is that it increases our cortisol production at the expense of progesterone. This leads to relative estrogen dominance because there isn't enough progesterone around to go head-to-head with estrogen. It's taken me many years to make my well-being a priority and my health has suffered as a result. These days I make time to destress with daily exercise and transcendental meditation, and I chant two times a day as part of my Nichirin Buddhist practice. As I was writing this book, I spoke to many, many women who are in perimenopause or just prior to perimeno-pause and 95 percent of them told me they were stressed. One of them even said: "I'm too stressed to deal with my stress!" The last thing I want to do is add to your stress. I'll just say you deserve to take time for yourself and to find ways to calm your body and mind. We all do!

- **Eat more fiber!** We have a fiber crisis in our country today. Okay, that may be an exaggeration, but we don't eat enough fiber and fiber is key to removing toxins from our bodies. Estrogen is processed by the liver and ideally should be excreted in our bowel movements, but if you aren't having regular bowel movements, estrogen is circulated back into your system. You want to aim for 145 grams of fiber per 1,000 calories. If you eat about 2,500 calories a day you should eat 35 grams of fiber each day. My favorite ways to get fiber are pumpkin seeds in my yogurt or smoothies, brown or forbidden rice with lunch or dinner, beans a couple of times a week and fruits and vegetables with every meal. Avocados have 10 grams of fiber per serving and oatmeal has 11 grams of fiber per serving. At a minimum, add these into your diet multiple times a week. If 14 grams of fiber per 1,000 calories is not possible for you given your current diet, add in a fiber supplement. Just go slowly for all the reasons you can imagine.

- **Move and sweat.** I talk about this is in greater detail in Chapter 11, so I'll just say here that exercise helps our bodies break down estrogen. Premenopausal women who engage in aerobic exercise for five hours a week or more saw their estrogen levels drop by nearly 19 percent. Cardiovascular exercise helps the body break estrogen down and flush away any excess.[25] If you are time strapped, you can achieve those five hours by working out in fifteen-minute increments if you prefer. The most important thing is to get it done and to sweat it out! If there's any chance that you may be estrogen dominant, committing to exercising until you sweat five hours week will help.

---

25 Smith, Alma J et al. "The effects of aerobic exercise on estrogen metabolism in healthy premenopausal women." *Cancer epidemiology, biomarkers & prevention: A publication of the American Association for Cancer Research, co-sponsored by the American Society of Preventive Oncology* vol. 22,5 (2013): 756–764. doi:10.1158/1055-9965.EPI-12-1325

Tracking your well-being, including symptoms, will give you a hint as to whether you are estrogen dominant and testing your hormones will provide confirmation. Go to www.helloperiwinkle.com/tracker to download our Well-Being Tracker.

- **Take DIM.** DIM, otherwise known as diindolylmethane, is a plant nutrient found in vegetables like cabbage, broccoli, bok choy, brussels sprouts and cauliflower. DIM has been a game changer for me because it helps create a pathway for estrogen to be metabolized in our bodies, which for me has meant reducing the symptoms associated with estrogen dominance. There is also research that shows that DIM can help with metabolizing estrogen.[26] I take the **Smoky Mountain Naturals** brand. Eating certain foods can also help with metabolizing estrogen and I go into greater detail about that in Chapter 9.

- **Take Calcium d-glucarate.** Calcium d-glucarate helps ensure estrogen marked for excretion actually leaves the body by inhibiting beta-glucaronidase from recycling the estrogen.[27] Without sufficient levels of calcium D-glucarate, estrogen can be activated and reabsorbed in the body, which means the liver then has to work again on clearing the reintroduced hormone, which strains the liver.

---

26 Lord RS, Bongiovanni B, Bralley JA. Estrogen metabolism and the diet-cancer connection: Rationale for assessing the ratio of urinary hydroxylated estrogen metabolites. Altern Med Rev. 2002 Apr;7(2):112–129. PMID: 11991791.

27 Calcium-D-glucarate. Altern Med Rev. 2002 Aug;7(4):336–339. PMID: 12197785.

Research[28] shows that supplementing with Calcium d-glucarate can assist the body in eliminating estrogen.

IMPORTANT NOTE 1: Because calcium d-glucarate can speed up the metabolism of toxins, it can also decrease the effectiveness of any medications you are taking. Talk with your care team before taking calcium d-glucarate. If after talking to your care team you decide to take calcium d-glucarate, you might want to take it a few hours away from your medication(s).

IMPORTANT NOTE 2: I have included in this chapter three herbal supplements that have helped me with estrogen dominance. Please note that all bodies are different and herbal supplements are not monitored by the FDA the same way medications are. You can't always be certain of what you're getting and whether it's safe. Herbal supplement contents may not be consistent and may include other ingredients. Remember, natural doesn't always mean safe. If you choose to take a supplement, please do so after doing your own research, choose supplements that have been third party tested and please let all of your healthcare providers know about all supplements you take.

---

28   Oredipe OA, Barth RF, Dwivedi C, Webb TE. Dietary glucarate-mediated inhibition of initiation of diethylnitrosamine-induced hepatocarcinogenesis. Toxicology. 1992 Sep;74(2-3):209–222. doi: 10.1016/0300-483x(92)90140-a. PMID: 1519243.

Chapter 7:

_____

HORMONE REPLACEMENT THERAPY: A LONG AND COMPLICATED STORY!

HORMONE REPLACEMENT THERAPY HAS changed my life. I was miserable two years ago: I never slept, I had hot flashes multiple times a day and I was anxious and irritable all the time. This had been going on for a couple of years. I tried everything: changed my diet, tried different exercise routines and started meditating, but nothing helped. My sister suggested I see a doctor who specializes in perimenopause and menopause, and she started me on progesterone and a small dose of estrogen. It took a couple of tries to get the right dosage and although I started out using an estrogen patch, I ended up using a cream instead. My sleep and irritability improved almost immediately and the hot flashes stopped soon after. I wish I hadn't suffered so long, and I wish more women knew that there are options for many of us. — *Shelly*

Now that you know hormone imbalances cause the physical and emotional symptoms we may experience in perimenopause, it stands to reason that the way to feel good and thrive in perimenopause is to balance our hormones.[29] This means we need to test our hormone levels to get a baseline and then test regularly thereafter. Once we know our levels, the goal is to address any imbalances. From my research, I have learned there are three options in perimenopause for addressing hormone imbalances:

OPTION 1: RIDE IT OUT

As you read earlier, 25 percent of women experience no perimenopause symptoms. If you are one of those women, you may not even know you are in perimenopause: lucky you! Some women may experience only one or two minor symptoms and may feel the symptoms are not problematic enough to treat. If you are one of those women, you may want to ride out the perimenopause stage and do nothing. This is a very valid option that I support with one caveat: if you do end up having symptoms later in menopause, it is important to understand that synthetic hormone replacement therapy becomes less of an option the older you get.

It is advised that women begin synthetic hormone replacement therapy either before age sixty or within ten years of the beginning of menopause. In other words, if my last menstrual cycle is in May at age forty-nine then I am officially in menopause in May the year I turn fifty, after one year without a period. This means I need to begin synthetic hormone replacement before May of the year I turn sixty. Please continue reading for detailed information on synthetic hormone replacement later in this chapter.

---

29 www.webmd.com/menopause/guide/menopause-hormone-therapy

OPTION 2: LIFESTYLE CHANGES AND HERBAL REMEDIES

As you read the remainder of this guide you will see that I dedicate an enormous amount of space and attention to specific strategies you can take to support your body and mind in perimenopause. Specifically, I include guidance on sleep, stress, alcohol use, foods that promote hormone balance and ways to move your body to support health and well-being. My hope is that these chapters will be helpful to you, and I encourage you to read them closely, take notes and apply the strategies you think will work for you in this time of life.

In addition to these suggestions, because some women prefer natural options to medications, which I go into detail about later in this chapter, I include guidance regarding herbs and vitamins you may wish to use during perimenopause to address hormone imbalance symptoms. Depending on the severity of your symptoms and specific imbalances, these herbs and vitamins may be helpful. I am not a health-care clinician, nor am I an herbalist, so please do your own research, work with your care team and always tell your care team about any and all herbs and vitamins you take.

Herbs and Vitamins

For Low Estrogen

- Research shows Vitamin E can help with hot flashes.[30]

- Black cohosh is a woodland herb native to North America. Some research shows black cohosh (when mixed with

---

30   Ziaei S, Kazemnejad A, Zareai M. The effect of vitamin E on hot flashes in menopausal women. Gynecol Obstet Invest. 2007;64(4):204–207. doi: 10.1159/000106491. Epub 2007 Jul 30. PMID: 17664882.

mixed with other herbals, Rheum rhaponticum and French maritime pine bark) can help with hot flashes.[31]

For Low Progesterone

- Vitamin C and Chasteberry (sometimes called Vitex) both support progesterone production. I took chasteberry early in perimenopause with success; however, in later perimenopause chasteberry was no longer effective and I began using bioidentical progesterone.

- Over-the-counter progesterone creams are also effective in early perimenopause.

The chasteberry plant, also called the chaste tree, is native to the Mediterranean region and Asia. Research indicates it helps with symptoms of PMS and breast pain associated with the menstrual cycle.[32]

For Low Testosterone

- Research shows zinc can increase testosterone levels in women. The research was done on women in menopause,

---

31 Ismail R, Taylor-Swanson L, Thomas A, Schnall JG, Cray L, Mitchell ES, Woods NF. Effects of herbal preparations on symptom clusters during the menopausal transition. Climacteric. 2015 Feb;18(1):11–28. doi: 10.3109/13697137.2014.900746. Epub 2014 Jul 4. PMID: 24605800.

32 Wuttke W, Jarry H, Christoffel V, Spengler B, Seidlová-Wuttke D. Chaste tree (Vitex agnus-castus): Pharmacology and clinical indications. Phytomedicine. 2003 May;10(4):348–357. doi: 10.1078/094471103322004866. PMID: 12809367.

but my sense is that it can be helpful in perimenopause as well.[33]

- Fenugreek is a plant belonging to the *Fabaceae* family and research indicates supplementing with Fenugreek can increase testosterone levels and sexual desire.[34] In addition to these suggestions, please look back at Chapter 6, and Chapters 11, 13 and 15 for additional vitamin and herbal remedies that can be helpful in supporting hormones during perimenopause.

OPTION 3: HORMONE REPLACEMENT THERAPY USING SYNTHETICS OR BIOIDENTICAL HORMONES

Many of us experience significant physical and emotional symptoms during perimenopause. For some of us, those symptoms interfere with our sleep, overall well-being, relationships, ability to exercise, sex lives and careers. I knew I needed to address the many ways my imbalanced hormones were affecting my life. Here's the thing: I had no idea hormone replacement therapy (HRT) was even an option. In fact, I believed HRT was incredibly dangerous! More on that later in this guide.

What Is Hormone Replacement Therapy?

---

33   Mazaheri Nia L, Iravani M, Abedi P, Cheraghian B. Effect of Zinc on Testosterone Levels and Sexual Function of Postmenopausal Women: A Randomized Controlled Trial. J Sex Marital Ther. 2021;47(8):804-813. doi: 10.1080/0092623X.2021.1957732. Epub 2021 Jul 27. PMID: 34311679.

34   Rao A, Steels E, Beccaria G, Inder WJ, Vitetta L. Influence of a Specialized Trigonella foenum-graecum Seed Extract (Libifem), on Testosterone, Estradiol and Sexual Function in Healthy Menstruating Women: A Randomised Placebo Controlled Study. Phytother Res. 2015 Aug;29(8):1123–1130. doi: 10.1002/ptr.5355. Epub 2015 Apr 24. PMID: 25914334.

As you learned in the previous chapters, during perimenopause our progesterone and estrogen levels decrease and also fluctuate quite a bit. Testosterone levels gradually decrease as we age. At age forty, our testosterone levels have lowered by half. Women who have had their ovaries surgically removed, women whose adrenal glands are not functioning properly and women who experience pituitary issues may experience low testosterone at an even earlier age. Many medications, including birth control pills, lower testosterone levels. DHEA and oxytocin levels also decrease with age. Hormone replacement therapy is the medication that replaces the estrogen, progesterone, testosterone, DHEA or oxytocin our bodies make less of in perimenopause and menopause.

Isn't Hormone Replacement Therapy Dangerous?

When I was in early perimenopause it never occurred to me to do HRT because I thought it was dangerous. I remembered that a number of studies in the 1990s and early 2000s showed HRT increased a woman's risk of cancer. As it turns out, things were more complicated than that. I feel like the backstory here is important so I'm going to share some history with you.[35]

As I shared earlier in this guide, stigmas associated with perimenopause exist today and the medical community still lacks adequate awareness and training in women's reproductive and sexual health beyond pregnancy. This is the case despite the fact that in the 1960s, with the rise of the feminist movement, there was a push to address women's health issues, including menopause. Menopausal therapy was encouraged, especially in Europe, and the best-selling

---

35   Cagnacci, Angelo, and Martina Venier. "The Controversial History of Hormone Replacement Therapy." *Medicina (Kaunas, Lithuania)* vol. 55,9 602. 18 Sep. 2019, doi:10.3390/medicina55090602

book *Feminine Forever*, published in 1966, asserted that estrogen supplementation should be used to address "hormone deficiencies." This was the beginning of an upswing in the use of estrogen replacement therapy. However, in the 1970s new studies were released showing that supplementing with estrogen by itself could lead to increased risk of endometrial cancer.[36] Researchers, however, continued to test hormone replacement options and found they could reduce the risk of endometrial cancer by decreasing the dose of estrogen and combining it with progesterone.[37] This makes total sense to me knowing estrogen and progesterone work in balance with one another!

Initially HRT was only approved by the FDA to treat hot flashes, but by 1988 it had been approved to prevent osteoporosis.[38] Over time clinicians expanded the use of HRT and began to prescribe HRT to prevent chronic diseases, including cardiovascular disease. Then, in 1998, the Women's Health Initiative (WHI) was launched. The WHI was a large, randomized study to look at the effect of HRT on the most common causes of death of older women—for example, cancer, cardiovascular disease and osteoporosis. The results of the study came out in 2002 and all heck broke loose.

---

36   4. Ziel H.K., Finkle W.D. Increased risk on endometrial carcinoma among users of conjugated estrogens. *N. Engl. J. Med.* 1975;293:1167–1170. doi: 10.1056/NEJM197512042932303.

37   Woodruff J.D., Pickar J.H. Incidence of endometrial hyperplasia in postmenopausal women taking conjugated estrogens (Premarin) with medroxyprogesterone acetate or conjugated estrogens alone. The Menopause Study Group. *Am. J. Obstet. Gynecol.* 1994;170:1213–1223. doi: 10.1016/S0002-9378(13)90437-3.

38   North American Menopause Society The 2012 hormone therapy position statement of the North American Menopause Society. *Menopause.* 2012;19:257–271. doi: 10.1097/gme.0b013e31824b970a.

Not only did the WHI study blow up the belief that HRT protected women from heart disease and other chronic illnesses, the research also said combining estrogen and progesterone increased a woman's risk of heart disease and breast cancer. The message women heard loud and clear was: "HRT is dangerous". I was 30 years old at the time the WHI study was released. I had a one-year-old baby and perimenopause was the last thing on my mind, but I remember clearly thinking to myself: "I need to remember this when I get older. I need to avoid HRT." As it turns out, I was not the only one thinking that way. Not surprisingly, the use of HRT decreased big time.

This is where things get interesting. Several factors related to the WHI study were not made clear at the time to women and to many in the medical community. Even today, there is confusion about the study. Here are three factors about the study that are important to know:

- First, the women in the WHI study were on average sixty-three years old, which is about twelve years older than the average age of menopause, fifty-one. This means very few of the patients were experiencing the symptoms HRT would be prescribed for in the first place. Additionally, because these patients were significantly older than women entering menopause, they also had multiple health issues than people who are older experience. About 35 percent of them were overweight, 34 percent were obese, 36 percent were hypertensive. Nearly 50 percent reported a history of smoking.[39] It's very possible the health status and age of the patients contributed to the results of the study.

---

39 Langer RD, White E, Lewis CE, Kotchen JM, Hendrix SL, Trevisan M. The Women's Health Initiative Observational Study: Baseline Characteristics of Participants and Reliability of Baseline Measures. Ann Epidemiol 2003;13:S107–S121. www.whi.org/about/Baseline%20Monograph/baseline_ObservationalStudy.pdf

- Second, the study researchers emphasized *relative risk* when speaking about breast cancer in the study:[40] *"The 26% increase (38 vs 30 per 10 000 person-years) observed in the estrogen plus progestin group **almost** reached nominal statistical significance and, as noted herein, the weighted test statistic used for monitoring was highly significant."* (**Note:** I have added the emphasis here.)

Absolute risk is your risk of developing a disease over a period of time. Relative risk is used to compare the risk in two different groups of people—for example, smokers versus nonsmokers. The emphasis on relative risk led to the belief that HRT causes breast cancer when, in fact, when you drill down into the research, you find that the *absolute risk* of breast cancer was increased in the estrogen-plus-progestin group by only eight breast cancer cases out of ten thousand women. That's an absolute increase of 0.08%, a much, much smaller risk than 26 percent. Not only that, but the 26 percent increase in relative risk *was not statistically significant.*

- Third, the women in the WHI were given Premarin, which was made from the urine of pregnant horses. In other words, the women in the study were given a kind of estrogen that is very different from that of human females.

I have gone into all these details about HRT and the WHI study because there are many women—and clinicians even—who continue to believe the WHI study determined HRT is dangerous and that the WHI study is the absolute last word on HRT. That is *not* the case. In

---

40 https://worldlinkmedical.com/what-you-need-to-know-about-the-womens-health-initiative

fact, since the WHI study, subsequent research has identified several important findings, including:[41]

- Hormone replacement therapy benefits younger women and those close to menopause, including protecting them against coronary disease. In other words, if HRT is given early enough (before age sixty and within ten years of menopause), it can be beneficial.

- The chances of strokes or blood clots in younger women who use HRT are so low they are called "rare" by the World Health Organization.

- Breast cancer rates are low with HRT use, and they are decreased when estrogen is used alone.

The disappointing part for me in sharing this background is that in the nearly twenty years since the WHI study, many, many women have suffered with perimenopause and menopause symptoms because they believed they had no options. These women had (have!) significant symptoms and yet they are either too scared to do HRT or their clinicians refuse to treat them with HRT. This decline in HRT use is largely due to a flawed study that has been widely misinterpreted.

The reality is that despite the WHI study and the overall decline in HRT use, many, many women (and men!) benefit greatly from HRT. I am personally one of those people and I recommend HRT to everyone I know. If you decide to do HRT, there are two routes you can take: synthetics and bioidenticals. Details on both are next.

---

41   Cagnacci, Angelo, and Martina Venier. "The Controversial History of Hormone Replacement Therapy." *Medicina* (Kaunas, Lithuania) vol. 55,9 602. 18 Sep. 2019, doi:10.3390/medicina55090602.

Hormone Replacement Options

There are two kinds of hormone replacement options. *Bioidentical* hormones are created in a laboratory and are typically plant based. *Synthetic* hormones are also made in a laboratory, and they are made from synthetic or manufactured materials. I provide detailed information about synthetic and bioidentical hormones in the next chapter.

Hormone Replacement Is an Option for Many Women!

What Kinds of Hormones Are –Available?

Numerous kinds of hormones available for HRT. They are described in what follows.

Estrogen Therapy Alone

- Estrogen therapy on its own is recommended for women who are done menstruating (technically in menopause) and who have undergone a hysterectomy and do not have a uterus. Estrogen requires a prescription.

- Estrogen therapy can be taken orally or via patches you put on your skin, sprays, gels or vaginal preparations. Estrogen therapy can also be given via pellets inserted under the skin. Some clinicians avoid prescribing oral estrogen because it passes through the liver as it is metabolized.

- Estrogen therapy is the best treatment for hot flashes, night sweats, brain fog, urinary issues, mood swings, depression, migraines, heart palpitations, vaginal flexibility and vaginal dryness.

IMPORTANT NOTE: IT is advised that women who are pregnant, have heart disease, a history of fibroids or blood clots, vaginal bleeding, gall bladder disease, liver disease and some types of estrogen-sensitive cancers not take estrogen. Estrogen must be prescribed by a doctor. Please work with your care team to determine whether it is safe for you to take estrogen.

Progesterone Therapy Alone

- Progesterone therapy alone (Progestin is the synthetic version) is recommended for women in perimenopause experiencing anxiety, sleep issues, irritability, sore breasts and heavy periods.

- Progesterone therapy can be taken orally or via cream. Over-the-counter creams can be effective in early peri-menopause but, toward the end of perimenopause as you get closer to menopause, you will likely need a prescription for oral or topical progesterone.

- *Note:* Progesterone can make you sleepy, so I take mine at night.

- In some cases progesterone and progestin are taken daily and clinicians prescribe them for only ten days prior to getting your period.

Combined Hormone Therapy

- If you still have a uterus, your doctor may prescribe combined hormone therapy. This is estrogen and progesterone (synthetic version is called progestin) taken together.

- Combined hormone therapy can help with hot flashes, vaginal dryness, sleep problems, urinary tract infections and other urinary issues and sore breasts.

- Research shows combined HRT can also lower our risk of colon cancer[42] and diabetes.[43]

- Combined hormone therapy can be taken orally, via patches or cream, via pellets inserted under the skin or via a ring inserted into the vagina.

- From the research I've done it appears that best route when it comes to taking estrogen (when you have a uterus) is to always take it with progesterone and use the lowest possible dose of estrogen that helps with symptoms for the shortest period of time possible.

- <u>Testosterone Hormone Therapy</u>

- Testosterone hormone therapy is recommended for women in perimenopause experiencing fatigue, brain fog, muscle loss, vaginal dryness, decreased motivation or depression.

- Testosterone hormone therapy for women is typically given via pellets inserted under the skin to avoid being metabolized via the liver, although some women replace

---

42 Rennert, Gad et al. "Use of hormone replacement therapy and the risk of colorectal cancer." *Journal of clinical oncology: Official journal of the American Society of Clinical Oncology* vol. 27,27 (2009): 4542–4547. doi:10.1200/JCO.2009.22.0764

43 Manning PJ, Allum A, Jones S, Sutherland WHF, Williams SM. The Effect of Hormone Replacement Therapy on Cardiovascular Risk Factors in Type 2 Diabetes: A Randomized Controlled Trial. *Arch Intern Med*.2001;161(14):1772–1776. doi:10.1001/archinte.161.14.1772

testosterone via injections. Testosterone cream can also be applied to the skin.

Oxytocin Replacement Therapy

- Oxytocin replacement therapy is recommended for women in perimenopause who have decreased sexual desire, are struggling to orgasm, have hypothyroidism or high cortisol levels or are experiencing depression or anxiety.

- Oxytocin replacement therapy can be taken as a nasal spray, as a sublingual tablet, topically as a cream or as an injection.

DHEA Replacement Therapy

- DHEA replacement therapy is recommended for women in perimenopause who have decreased sexual desire or depressed mood.

IMPORTANT NOTE: In the United States, testosterone replacement has been FDA approved only for men, not for women, and is only available as a bioidentical hormone. However, this is true for many drugs that are still widely prescribed and used. In the United States, oxytocin replacement therapy has not been FDA approved and is only available as bioidentical hormones.

I would like to offer to you, dear reader, several pieces of guidance based on my experience with HRT:

- It is very important to work with a care team that checks your hormone levels regularly, especially before you receive a new dose of a medicine. For example, my care team checks my testosterone levels each time before I receive testosterone replacement therapy. This is important to ensure that you are receiving appropriate doses. The majority of women I have spoken with who have experienced side effects from HRT have experienced symptoms because their care team is not testing their hormone levels regularly.

- Even after you begin HRT it is important to track your well-being. Perimenopause is a journey and our hormones can shift even with and during HRT. Tracking your well-being and taking note of specific symptoms or side affects you are experiencing will help your care team decide the best way to manage those symptoms and side effects. Download our Well-Being Tracker at helloperiwinkle.com/tracker

A Word about Bioidentical and Synthetic Hormones

As I was doing the research for this guide, I found strong opinions and conflicting information when it comes to bioidentical and synthetic hormones. For example:

- Some people, including many functional medicine and integrative medicine clinicians, believe bioidentical hormones are a better option compared to synthetic hormones because they consider them more natural (note there is in-depth information about functional medicine and integrative medicine clinicians in the next chapter).

- Some people, including many mainstream clinicians, believe bioidentical hormones are not, in fact, more natural because while they are created from plants, they are combined with other synthetic materials.

- Some people, including many functional medicine and integrative clinicians, are wary of synthetic hormones, pointing to medications like Prempro, which was a combination of two drugs containing synthetic hormones, which caused cancer and heart disease in many women.

- Some people, including many mainstream clinicians, only prescribe synthetic hormones because they are unaware of bioidenticals or believe they are not as effective as synthetic hormones.

- To complicate things even more, some bioidentical hormones are premade by drug companies while others are custom-made by a pharmacist based on a doctor's order. This is known as compounding. There are numerous FDA bioidentical hormones, but the compounded forms have not been tested and approved by the FDA. However, according to the North American Menopause Society (NAMS), about 1.4 million women use compounded treatments yearly. That's because thousands of clinicians write prescriptions for non-FDA approved medications every year. They also write prescriptions for off-label use, meaning the medication was created for one purpose but has proven effective for others. Just because a drug is not FDA approved does not make it automatically unsafe.

With all of that said, my research into bioidenticals versus synthetics uncovered one piece of information I believe is important to share with you. There are two versions of progesterone: the bioidentical version is called Prometrium and the synthetic version is called Provera. Both are FDA approved; however, studies on Provera have shown that women have many more side effects from Provera.

I believe we all need to make our own decisions when it comes to choosing bioidentical and synthetic hormones. Please supplement what I have shared here with your own research and then find a care team to talk to and ask questions to learn more. The next chapter is all about finding your perimenopause dream team!

Chapter 8:

THE PERIMENOPAUSE DREAM TEAM

"NONE OF MY DOCTORS EVER ASKED ME IF I was experiencing perimenopause symptoms. None of them warned me ahead of time about what I should expect. I'm most disappointed in my obstetrician-gynecologist. She watched me suffer with postpartum depression with both of my pregnancies but never once asked if I was struggling because of hormone shifts. She never mentioned the potential of experiencing emotional or mental health challenges. Worst of all she blew off my concerns about not sleeping." — *Marilyn*

Twenty-one years ago when my husband and I decided we wanted to start a family I asked friends and family members for recommendations of obstetricians and pediatricians. I met with several clinical teams and finally chose practices where I felt like the clinicians would meet my needs and my future children's needs. For example, I decided against one obstetrics practice because they refused to allow doulas to attend births. I also remember clearly knocking one pediatrician out of the running when she told me she believed all children should be at home with parents or a nanny and said disparaging things about day care centers (we preferred day care settings for our kids. Your mileage may vary.). Ultimately, I was fortunate in that I was cared for by a caring team of obstetricians and my children and my husband and I forged a long-term relationship with a knowledgeable and caring team of pediatricians.

Interestingly, despite being a natural "planner" and despite knowing the health-care system well due to my career, it never occurred to me to ask for referrals or to vet health-care providers in my late thirties, early forties as I entered perimenopause. I wish I could go back in time and ask myself what I was thinking. I can only imagine I was very busy managing my business and my family's needs and I naively assumed everything would be fine. You know by now that was not the case for me.

Please Begin Planning Now!

If you are reading this book and you have not yet entered perimeno-pause or you are very early in perimenopause, *right now* is the perfect time to start thinking about the care you want to receive in perimeno-pause and the kind of care team who will give you the right care. If you are currently in perimenopause, it doesn't mean it's too late to put together your perimenopause dream team. Take it from me: it's never too late to make your health and well-being a priority. Like anything else, a little leg work and preparation will pay off in the long run.

WHAT TO LOOK FOR

When looking for your perimenopause dream team keep in mind that certain things should be nonnegotiable. A dream team will:

- Get to know you as a person.

- Listen to your needs.

- Work to understand how you're feeling physically, emotionally *and* mentally.

- Ask you about your symptoms and how long you've had them.

- View you as a whole person and not just a collection of body parts.

- Take labs regularly to monitor your hormone levels, including and especially your thyroid.

- Share knowledge and information about addressing perimenopause symptoms.

- Offer a range of options for addressing your perimenopause symptoms.

- Help you identify cost-effective options.

- Partner with you in all aspects of your health-care decision-making while also recognizing that ultimately the decisions are yours to make.

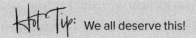 **Hot Tip:** We all deserve this!

SPECIALIZATION IS IMPORTANT

I feel very strongly about the advice I'm about to share and I feel like it's only fair to give you a heads up. It may be controversial to some people, but I can't publish this guide without saying it. *Your peri-menopause dream team should be made up of clinicians who specialize in women's sexual and reproductive health and/or who specialize in hormone balancing.*

Perimenopause is all about hormones. That's the bottom line. Keeping those hormones in balance will define your perimenopause experience. By now, you have a good sense of all the hormones at play in our bodies and the ways in which they fluctuate in perimenopause. You also know keeping those hormones in balance can be a challenge. It's important to make sure the clinicians who care for you know every-thing there is to know about hormones. You want them to be deeply familiar with the research to date, tracking new research and studies and well-versed in the most-up-to-date treatments available, as well as the pros and cons of those treatments. I'm a firm believer that all of us in perimenopause should work with a team that is passionate about women's hormones and committed to supporting women to achieve their best health and wellness in their midlife.

FINDING A DREAM TEAM CAN BE TOUGH

Here's the thing: finding a perimenopause dream team is not as simple as finding a pediatrician or gynecologist. You cannot assume most—or even the majority—of health care clinicians are experts in hormones and women's sexual health. Far from it! In fact, in a 2017 survey of medical residents in family medicine, internal medicine and obstetrics and gynecology, 20.3 percent reported not receiving any menopause lectures during residency, and only 6.8 percent reported feeling adequately prepared to manage women experiencing meno-pause.[44] Frustratingly, the survey doesn't even ask about perimeno-

---

44   www.mayoclinicproceedings.org/article/S0025-6196(18)30701-8/
     fulltext#articleInformation

pause, which is a problem, but regardless, the fact that only 6.8 percent of residents report feeling adequately prepared to care for women in menopause is incredibly disappointing.

I know I'm not alone in wanting a health-care team that has studied extensively the ins and outs of women's sexual and reproductive health and that has a long history of helping women identify and treat perimenopause symptoms. So, why don't most clinicians know as much about women's hormones and reproductive and sexual health as we'd like? There are a number of reasons:

- Medicine has been male dominated until very recently. As a result, women's health conditions have been under researched and underfunded. Did you know the FDA excluded "females of childbearing potential" from clinical trials from 1977 through 1993?[45] Even after the National Institutes of Health mandated the inclusion of women in clinical research, women's health continued to be overlooked. For example, although cardiovascular disease is the leading cause of death among women (and men) only one-third of cardiovascular clinical trial subjects have been female, and fewer than one-third of the trials that included women reported outcomes by sex. This means even the most well-meaning medical professionals can find themselves underinformed and ill-prepared to offer effective solutions and support to women regarding their health.

- No specific health-care clinician specialty has "owned" perimenopause or menopause. Therefore, you should not assume your gynecologist or your primary care clinician

45 www.fda.gov/science-research/womens-health-research/ regulations-guidance-and-reports-related-womens-health

will be a perimenopause expert. In fact, there's very little chance they are.

- In many cultures a stigma is associated with both women's health issues and women's sexual health issues. Stigmas are very powerful and affect all of us, even health-care professionals. Stigmas shut down conversation, content sharing and knowledge building. This means a lot of us are on our own when it comes to perimenopause.

TWO PATHWAYS

You have two pathways when it comes to finding a perimenopause dream team:

- **Pathway 1:** Work with your current clinician(s).

- **Pathway 2:** Find new clinicians.

Read on for specific guidance on both pathways.

Pathway 1

Step 1: Do not assume your current care team is knowledgeable about women's sexual health and reproductive issues or hormone balancing.

Step 2: Ask! You should inquire about your care team's experience with perimenopause, especially if you have a long-standing and trusting relationship with them. For example, if you have a well visit coming up to get a breast exam or pap smear, find out the specific knowledge and expertise your current care team has when it comes to women's sexual and reproductive health and hormone balancing. A good way to open the conversation is to say: *What is your experience helping women* *manage their hormone health? When do you start conversations about perimenopause with patients?*

Step 3: If they say they have experience, probe into how they help patients manage their perimenopause symptoms, using everything you learned in Chapters 3, 4 and 7.

Step 4: Ask them to test your hormones to get a baseline. If they refuse, find a different care team because knowing your hormone levels is key to managing perimenopause effectively.

Hot Tip: Do not assume your health care team will ask you about perimenopause. In fact, the many women I interviewed and surveyed for this book told me over and over that the overwhelming thing they received from their care team before and during perimenopause was silence. You need to be prepared to raise the issue.

IMPORTANT NOTE: If when you bring up perimenopause or hormones your clinician seems uncomfortable, minimizes your concern in anyway or prescribes birth control without checking your hormone levels, these are red flags that tell you they are not a dream team. Do not doubt yourself or ignore these signs!

Pathway 2:

You may find your current care team does not have the specialized knowledge or experience you would like to support you in perimenopause. If that's the case, there are multiple ways to find clinicians with this expertise. For example:

- Search online or with your health insurance plan for clinicians who specialize in women's sexual health, reproductive health (some fertility doctors also specialize in perimenopause and menopause care) or hormone balancing. Oftentimes a practice's website will include these exact phrases.

- Another option is to find a certified menopause practitioner via the North American Menopause Society (www. menopause.org/for-women/whats-an-ncmp). They will be helpful in navigating perimenopause and will also be available to you as you enter menopause.

- If you prefer to work with a care team that specializes in bioidentical HRT you can search by zip code and state for clinicians with that specialization at www.foreverhealth. com.

- Ask friends and family members or post on your community message boards. One of the ways we will reduce the stigma associated with perimenopause is to be transparent about our needs.

- Do research to find reproductive endocrinologists (details later). In writing this book I learned a growing number of reproductive endocrinologists are focusing on perimenopause and menopause.

- Look for functional and integrative medicine clinicians (details later). I have benefited greatly from working with functional and integrative medicine clinicians, and most people who know me personally have heard me extol the virtues of functional medicine.

Reproductive Endocrinology

Reproductive endocrinology is a medical specialty. Reproductive endocrinologists are OB/GYN (obstetrics and gynecology) doctors with special training to help both men and women with problems related to reproductive hormones. Sometimes this specialty is called reproductive endocrinology and infertility because much of their work focuses on helping women become pregnant and carry a baby to term. However, because these clinicians are well versed in hormones, some of them may be helpful in perimenopause and menopause. In fact, in my research I found that while these clinicians typically focus on infertility issues, a growing number of them are focusing on perimenopause and menopause. You can search for reproductive endocrinologists on these websites:

https://health.usnews.com/doctors/location-index/reproductive-endocrinologists; https://doctor.webmd.com/find-a-doctor/specialty/reproductive-endocrinology; www.healthgrades.com/fertility-reproductive-endocrinology-directory.

Functional and Integrative Medicine

Functional and integrative medicine clinicians are trained in traditional medicine, but the way they practice and the methods they use differ from traditional medicine. Importantly, functional medicine and integrative medicine clinicians are patient-centered rather than symptom-focused. In other words, they look at patients as a whole to understand the causes of symptoms and conditions rather than starting with symptoms. This means they look at the entirety of a patient's well-being: the physical, emotional, mental, societal and environmental factors that may be affecting a patient's health.

Many functional medicine and integrative medicine clinicians incorporate "alternative" or "integrative" medical techniques such as acupuncture and herbs into their treatment that are not typically used in traditional health care. Integrative medicine also focuses on the nutritional and exercise habits of patients and integrative medicine clinicians support patients in improving their personal habits to address chronic diseases, life stages or conditions. I am very supportive functional medicine and integrative medicine and have experienced only two downsides to functional and integrative medicine:

- There are fewer functional and integrative medicine practices than traditional medical practices, which means there may not be a practice in your town or community. However, as I write this guide, the health-care system has undergone many changes due to the COVID-19 pandemic and telehealth has become more accepted, so it's possible you can work with a functional or integrative medicine clinician from a distance using telehealth.

- Unfortunately, it can be challenging to find a functional or integrative medicine practice within many health insurance networks. In some cases, a visit may be covered but insurance will only cover a portion of the many labs that many functional or integrative medicine clinicians order. This makes functional or integrative medicine expensive for many people and completely out of reach for others. You can search for functional and integrative medicine clinicians on these websites: www.ifm.org/find-a-practitioner; https://integrativemedicine.arizona.edu/alumni.html

In talking with women in advance of writing this book I noticed some trends:

- Many women who go to mainstream clinicians in early perimenopause with symptoms are prescribed birth control pills (synthetic hormones) to manage their symptoms, frequently without having their specific hormones levels checked. To me, this is a one-size-fits-all approach.

- Many women who go to mainstream clinicians later in perimenopause, nearing menopause, are offered antidepressants. Note: antidepressants are *not* appropriate treatment for managing perimenopause or menopause symptoms. They may help with some of the anxiety and depression we experience in perimenopause, but they are masking the real issue, which is unbalanced hormones.

- Some of the women I spoke with were able to get their mainstream clinicians to prescribe synthetic hormones, but only after they brought up the subject and advocated for themselves. That's not surprising given that in a NAMS survey, only 57 percent of physicians were up to date on HRT information.

- A number of the women I spoke with were told by mainstream clinicians to stop drinking alcohol and caffeine, and that was the only guidance they were provided.

- On the flip side, I spoke with many women who partner with functional and integrative medicine clinicians during perimenopause. I am one of those people. These clinicians check hormone levels regularly, they are knowledgeable about HRT—while at the same time they share guidance on

how lifestyle choices can assist with hormone balancing—
and they aim for a personalized approach to addressing
hormone imbalances.

I did not write this guide in order to extol the virtues of functional
and integrative medicine clinicians, but I hope these observations and
sharing my personal experiences are helpful. Ultimately the decision
is yours to make.

IMPORTANT NOTE: As I wrote this guide I found many
"health coaches" and "functional medicine nutritionists" online.
While I believe strongly that we all need and deserve support
during perimenopause and menopause, and while I also believe
that nutrition and exercise can be key to effectively managing
perimenopause and menopause symptoms, I do not recommend
working with "health coaches" and "functional medicine
nutritionists" as a substitute for working with a clinician who can
test your hormones or who is trained to interpret hormone lab data
and make treatment recommendations according to those data.

My sincere hope is that by launching Periwinkle and by writing this
book I am doing my part to change our culture and our medical system
so women's sexual and reproductive health-care needs are viewed as a
priority. In an ideal world, over the course of the next decade (hopefully sooner!), the health-care system will recognize the health and
well-being of nearly one billion women worldwide matters, and there
will be less stigma associated with perimenopause and menopause
and greater transparency and support available. My greatest dream
is that we will see:

- Perimenopause and menopause curricula in medical schools and in residency.

- Increased knowledge and comfort among all clinicians about women's sexual and reproductive health, including hormone balancing.

- More clinicians providing women with actionable information before they are in perimenopause.

- A surge in gender- and sex-specific clinical trials aimed at better understanding how to help women manage perimenopause and menopause.

- Better treatment for perimenopause and menopause.

Chapter 9:

FOOD IS NOT THE ENEMY

> **"MY BIGGEST STRUGGLE IN PERIMENOPAUSE**
> was weight gain. I couldn't help but feel like everything I put
> in my mouth was causing me to gain weight, so I kept cutting
> back my calories only to end up cranky and frustrated. Basically,
> I demonized food. Late in perimenopause I started eating for
> hormone health and it changed everything. I now maintain a
> healthy weight without starving myself, and not surprisingly I'm a
> heck of a lot happier." — *Annick*

If there's anything I love as much as sleep, it's food. My mother is a
wonderful cook, and I am lucky enough to be married to a man who
is a phenomenal cook. Two of my hobbies are trying out new restau-
rants and traveling to places with foods I could never find at home.
Prior to perimenopause I ate healthfully most of the time, but beyond
making sure I ate lots of fruits and vegetables it never occurred me
to think of food as anything more than sustenance and enjoyment.
That's not to say I have not struggled with my weight. I gained fifty

pounds with both of my pregnancies and my weight has fluctuated throughout my life.

Perimenopause was a whole new ballgame, though. I gained twenty pounds overnight, struggled to move my body and experienced pain in my body most hours of the day. I needed help and, unfortunately, I began to view food as the enemy because everything I ate seemed to make me gain weight.

If you perused the table of contents for this guide you may have noticed it does not include a chapter on dieting or weight loss. Depending on what you're experiencing in perimenopause, or on your own history with weight and food intake, you may feel relieved or you may feel royally disappointed. Many women have told me it felt like their metabolism exited the building (their body!) as they entered perimenopause, leaving them with unwanted pounds and feeling unhappy with their bodies, and like me, they decided food was the problem. I get it!

However, there are lots of reasons you may be gaining weight, feeling bloated or seeing more fat and less muscle during perimenopause that have very little to do with what you are eating:

1. **Loss of Muscle Mass.** The average adult loses 3–8 percent of muscle during each decade after age thirty.[46] Muscle converts easily to fat as we age, and without muscle our bodies burn fewer calories at rest, while we sleep and when we exercise.

2. **Hormonal Changes.** Our estrogen levels start to fluctuate in perimenopause, so our bodies look for ways to replace

---

46   English, Kirk L, and Douglas Paddon-Jones. "Protecting muscle mass and function in older adults during bed rest." *Current opinion in clinical nutrition and metabolic care* vol. 13,1 (2010): 34–39. doi:10.1097/MCO.0b013e328333aa66

estrogen. Fat, which produces estrone, the weakest version of the three types of estrogen, is one option. This often results in new fat deposits, especially in our bellies.

3. **Dehydration.** Estrogen levels can impact our ability to regulate fluids. Because it takes more time for our bodies to replenish fluids, many of us end up experiencing low levels of dehydration. Water helps regulate body temperature, keeps joints lubricated and may also play a role in weight. According to some studies, the energy provided by water helps the body burn fat via lipolysis, the process by which the body burns fat for energy. Lack of hydration in the body decreases lipolysis.

4. **Thyroid Issues.** Your thyroid is in charge of your metabolic drive. If it's not working at the appropriate level, it's almost impossible to prevent weight gain. Check out Chapter 5 for more information about your thyroid.

5. **Too Much Cortisol.** Cortisol is our stress hormone. When we are stressed, our bodies release cortisol to raise our blood sugar levels, giving us energy to respond to whatever is causing us stress. In perimenopause many of us lack adequate progesterone levels to counteract high cortisol. High levels of cortisol can kick off a series of responses that can ultimately lead to obesity, which in turn can lead to heart disease, diabetes and sometimes death. Not good!

In other words, weight gain in perimenopause is about more than what we eat. Extreme diets are tempting when we feel like we're walking around in a body that isn't ours. On a practical level, it's frustrating when you've outgrown all of your clothes and the only way to avoid inappropriate nudity is to buy a new wardrobe. I admit, as I watched the scale move higher and higher during perimenopause, I felt myself becoming desperate. I started skipping meals. I looked into extreme diets. I added in more and more exercise. Take it from me, this is *not* the way to go. Sure, you may lose some weight quickly, but it's unlikely the weight will stay off, you may burn out your adrenal gland and, most importantly, you will deprive your body of important nutrients it needs now more than ever. In this chapter I'm going to share with you a three-step approach that will invite you to let go of any body or diet baggage you may be carrying around after more than thirty years on this planet and give you the nutrition your body needs in perimenopause.

STEP ONE: PLEASE BE KIND TO YOURSELF

I took a completely nonscientific poll of my female friends and acquaintances a couple of years ago. First, I asked them: "How do you feel about your body?"

- One hundred percent of them told me, "Not great."

- At least 60 percent of them went into great detail about what they were unhappy with and what they wanted to change:

  » "My hips are my nemesis. They've been too big since I was seventeen."

  » "Look at these bat wings! My arms are awful."

  » "It doesn't matter how much I exercise. My butt is flat and wide."

I could go on and on, but I'll spare you more details because the comments made me sad. Trust me, I'm not immune to these kinds of comments myself! When I gained weight during perimenopause I said horrible things to myself about my various body parts multiple times a day. News flash: beating up on yourself does not lead to body positivity. Speaking badly about our body erodes our self-esteem over time! Please don't do that to yourself.

The second question in my nonscientific poll was: "Have you ever been on a diet? If so, when was your first diet and why?" Here's what I learned:

- One hundred percent of the women I asked said yes, they had been on a diet in their lifetime.

- One hundred percent said their first diet was between ages thirteen and sixteen.

- One hundred percent of them said they went on a diet to lose weight.

Even from a totally nonscientific poll, these answers gave me pause. While it is true worldwide obesity has nearly tripled since 1975, the women I spoke with were teenagers in the 1980s and 1990s when obesity rates were much lower.[47] Could it be that they were raised in cultures that prioritize female "thinness" and encourage girls and women to go to extremes to reach unattainable bodies? I'm being facetious here: of course they were. *We have all been indoctrinated into diet culture—our children too!*

Culture Is Powerful

Many external messages conspire against us and lead us to criticize ourselves. Fashion magazines, Hollywood, social media etc. all include

---

47   www.who.int/news-room/fact-sheets/detail/obesity-and-overweight

unrealistic images of women that are impossible to attain. Diet culture is a huge industry and few of us are immune from its influence.

Unfortunately, this guide can't tackle dismantle the culture that makes us scrutinize our bodies (although I will find a way to do that someday!). This guide is not going to eliminate the cabbage soup diet, the cayenne pepper/honey diet, the bacon ten times a day diet or any other insane approach to eating. This guide is also not going to stop spam messages that offer quick fixes to address the extra pounds many of gain as we go through midlife and our hormones shift. We can take steps not to fall into the trap of trying to attain "perfect" bodies.

What You Can Do

I want to encourage *you* to leave behind the unfair expectations you have for *yourself*. If you're reading this guide, you're likely thirty-two years old or older. Isn't it time you stopped listening to the messages that tell you you're flawed and not enough? Are you going to go to your grave disappointed in your bat wings? Enough! I don't know you, but I know you are so much more than your thighs. The women I know are brilliant, resourceful, kind and hilarious. Not once have I ever thought about their bat wings!

The reason I'm harping on this *Be Kind to Yourself* step is because I've spent hours researching the Internet and it's a scary place teeming with "How to Lose Weight in Perimenopause" schemes all trying to capitalize on your fears and insecurities. The reality is:

1. There is nothing wrong with you.

2. It is completely *normal* to gain weight in perimenopause for all of the reasons outlined earlier in this chapter.

3. It is possible to be a healthy weight in perimenopause and menopause.

STEP TWO: TEST YOUR HORMONES

What can we do in perimenopause and menopause to achieve a healthy weight? If you've gotten this far in the guide, you know the main theme running throughout it is: balance your hormones. Balanced hormones are the difference between minor physical, mental and emotional changes in perimenopause and a full-on personal meltdown. So, *Step Two: Test Your Hormones and Find a Health-Care Team* that specializes in hormone balancing so they can support your health and well-being in perimenopause.

STEP THREE: EAT FOR HORMONE HEALTH

Let me be clear: food alone *cannot* balance your hormones. Period, end of story. I feel like I need to say that again or light off fireworks or something to underscore this point. Don't get me wrong. Nutrition is key to supporting your body through perimenopause. What you eat and drink will either aid in hormone health or it will deter your efforts to achieve hormone health. But it will not balance your hormones. So, let's dive in!

Foods to Prioritize

<u>Whole grains</u>

Adding whole grains to your diet, such as brown rice, wheat bread and oatmeal, makes us feel full, and whole grains give us the energy we need to get through the day. I suggest choosing grains that are high in fiber to help your internal and natural detox processes (aka poop!). Remember, we want to ensure estrogen leaves the body versus recirculating in the body, otherwise we become estrogen dominant. See Chapter 6 for more information about why regular bowel movements are important to hormone health.

Calcium-Rich Foods

Because our bones begin to weaken during perimenopause, adding calcium-rich foods to your diet will help build them back up. Aim for at least 1,000 mg of calcium per day. I make sure I eat one or two servings of foods such as yogurt, cheese, broccoli, canned sardines or salmon, almonds and kale every day. I am very concerned about the hormones and antibiotics given to many cows in the United States, so whenever possible I consume dairy products that are hormone and antibiotic free or I choose goat dairy products. Your mileage may vary.

Fat

I cannot emphasize enough that our bodies need fat at all times in our lives, but even more so in perimenopause as we are dealing with fluctuating hormones. We need fat to make hormones! Omega-3 fatty acids have a great reputation because they help with inflammation and improved mood, including decreasing depression, which is something many of us experience during perimenopause. You can get omega-3 fatty acids by eating fish a couple of times a week or by taking fish oil supplements. Flaxseed oil is another option if you are not estrogen dominant.

In addition to omega-3 fatty acids I make sure I eat butter and olive oil every day and I eat avocados and nuts and nut butters multiple times a week. It can be tempting to cut down on fat when we see our weight creeping up, but cutting fat in perimenopause just adds to the stress our bodies are already under and we end up creating more cortisol, leading to a vicious cycle.

Artichokes

Once our bodies use hormones, they have to get rid of them. The liver works to metabolize our hormones, which then get excreted in the urine and stool. Artichokes do a great job of supporting our liver function and are also high in fiber. Look back at Chapter 6 for more suggestions of foods that support your liver.

Protein

High-protein foods are rich in essential amino acids that facilitate the release of hormones that control our appetite. Foods high in protein also help regulate the hunger hormone ghrelin to make us feel less hungry and stimulate other hormones that make us feel full for longer periods of time. I don't eat red or white meat, but I make sure I get as close to my body's needs as per my body weight in protein grams daily through eggs, whey protein, beans, nuts and seafood. For example, a 150-pound woman should aim for 150 grams of protein a day. I found that prioritizing protein in perimenopause helped me enormously, especially since I lift weights and my body needs protein to build muscle.

While I am good about eating enough protein, I have found through trial and error that protein alone does not satisfy me, so I combine my protein with other foods. Here are some ideas to get you started:

- Hardboiled egg, piece of toast, an apple.

- Brown rice, roasted salmon, cabbage.

- Tuna fish, leafy greens, quinoa.

- Forbidden rice, black beans, peppers and onions.

Water

Our bodies tend toward dehydration during perimenopause. Among other reasons, many of us find ourselves sweating more than we ever have in our lives due to hot flashes and night sweats. This dehydration can lead to dizziness for some of us, and to dry skin, mouths etc. as well. We need to prioritize hydration, and water is the best way to do that. I suggest drinking one-half to two-thirds of your body weight in ounces of water each day. For example, someone who weighs 150 pounds should drink at least 75 ounces each day.

THINGS YOU MAY WANT TO AVOID

- **Caffeine.** Hot flashes can be exacerbated by caffeine, so give it up altogether, limit your caffeine intake or choose options with lower caffeine amounts like green tea and matcha.

- **Alcohol.** Alcohol can cause hot flashes and increase estrogen levels. See Chapter 10 for more information about alcohol and perimenopause.

- **Sugar.** As I mentioned earlier in this chapter, low estrogen levels often result in cravings for carbohydrates and sugar. The problem with giving in to these cravings is that when we eat sugar our insulin levels rise and our brain gets a "shot" of the dopamine, but now we associate sugar with feeling good and we create a cycle where we need/want and consume more sugar. Sugar is high in calories and low in nutrition and our bodies need nutritious food. In addition, sugar is empty calories, which we definitely don't need as our muscle mass is decreasing. Instead we need food like protein that promotes muscle growth.

Foods That May Help or Harm

Soy. I avoid soy (soy beans, edamame, tofu, tempeh, natto, miso etc.) except for rare occasions. Soy is a plant protein containing phytoestrogens (hormones derived from plants) called isoflavones, which have an estrogen-like structure. Soy isoflavones either stimulate or block estrogen response. If you think you, like me, are estrogen dominant or you have tested your hormones and the test has confirmed estrogen dominance, this means soy could increase your estrogen levels if consumed regularly. On the other hand, if you are low in estrogen, soy could help stave off hot flashes and other symptoms, which is the case in Japan, for example, where women rarely experience perimenopause or menopause symptoms. My other concern with soybeans is that they are the number one genetically modified food crop in the world and treated extensively with pesticides. If you have concerns about this (I do!), I suggest avoiding soy products.

Some Seeds (flax and sesame). Flaxseeds are filled with lignans, a group of chemical compounds that functions as phytoestrogens. In fact, flaxseeds contain up to eight hundred times more lignans than other plant foods.[48] Sesame seeds are also quite rich in phytoestrogens. Similar to soy, these phytoestrogens can be problematic if you are estrogen dominant, but they can be helpful if you are not.

A FINAL THOUGHT

I began this chapter by encouraging you not to demonize food and to release yourselves from the brainwashing many of us have been

---

48   Bergman Jungeström M, Thompson LU, Dabrosin C. Flaxseed and its lignans inhibit estradiol-induced growth, angiogenesis, and secretion of vascular endothelial growth factor in human breast cancer xenografts in vivo. Clin Cancer Res. 2007 Feb 1;13(3):1061–1067. doi: 10.1158/1078-0432.CCR-06-1651. PMID: 17289903.

exposed to about needing to be thin. I hope this chapter has convinced you there are many normal and natural reasons our bodies (and our weight) change in perimenopause. We are doing nothing wrong. We do, however, have control over what how we think about ourselves, whether we address our hormones and what we eat. I encourage you to look at food differently from here on out. It's definitely not the enemy. In fact, lot of food is delicious and it's often the way we bring friends and family together, and it can also be a tool for helping us manage hormone health. Salut!

Chapter 10:

THE TRUTH ABOUT ALCOHOL
AND PERIMENOPAUSE

> **"I HAVE FOUND MYSELF TURNING TO WINE**
> at night more than I ever have in my life. I think it's because I'm
> so anxious. I need a way to unwind and turn off my brain. I also
> have such a hard time falling asleep at night that I end up drinking
> two or three glasses of wine to knock myself out. Unfortunately,
> it doesn't help me stay asleep. I've been waking up at 4:00 a.m.
> for months now." — *Amy*

As you've read through this guide so far, you've likely noticed a very
prominent theme: thriving during perimenopause and, ultimately,
during menopause itself, comes down to testing your hormones, balancing them, testing them again and repeating. That's because in perimenopause hormones are shifting all of the time, which results in some
hormones being below ideal levels and others above ideal levels. One
of the things to keep in mind is that alcohol can affect our hormones.
It's important before or during perimenopause to:

- Examine your relationship with alcohol.

- Understand the ways in which alcohol affects your hormones.

- Create strategies to either reduce or eliminate alcohol if it is affecting your hormones.

Estrogen and Alcohol

Bottom line—and not great news if you like a cocktail—alcohol affects how we metabolize estrogen. In fact, alcohol increases the amount of estrogen in our blood.[49] This is a problem because we want our hormones to be in balance and we definitely want to avoid estrogen dominance! Not only that, but these higher estrogen levels may increase our risk of breast cancer.[50]

Testosterone and Women and Alcohol

As I described in earlier chapters, testosterone is an important hormone, not just for men but for women too. Testosterone helps with building muscle and tissues, protein synthesis and increasing bone density. For women in particular, the maintenance of bone density and muscle mass is important, as they both tend to deteriorate as we age. The other reasons testosterone is important to women are mood, energy levels and sexual desire. Testosterone is the "feel good" hormone. When it's at the right level it gives us energy and sustains our sexual desire. When it's lower than ideal, we can feel depressed.

---

49 Jan Gill, The effects of moderate alcohol consumption on female hormone levels and reproductive function, *Alcohol and Alcoholism*, Volume 35, Issue 5, September 2000, Pages 417–423, https://doi.org/10.1093/alcalc/35.5.417

50 www.komen.org/breast-cancer/facts-statistics/research-studies/how-to-read-a-research-table/#pooled-analyses

Unfortunately, many of us aren't aware of how important testosterone is to our well-being or what we need to do to ensure healthy testosterone levels.

Changes in Testosterone Levels over Time

For women ages nineteen and older, normal testosterone levels range from 8 to 60 ng/dL, according to Mayo Clinic Laboratories. This is approximately one-tenth to one-twentieth of the normal levels of testosterone in men. Testosterone levels peak when we are teens and decrease as we age.

A small percentage of women (4–7 percent) produce too much testosterone in their ovaries. Some of these women have polycystic ovary syndrome (PCOS). Other possible effects of high testosterone levels in women are excessive hair growth in unwanted areas, acne, excessive perspiration, frontal balding and deepening of the voice.

In perimenopause, we are much more likely to experience low testosterone than high. That's because, again, testosterone levels decrease over time and because many women tend to be estrogen dominant during perimenopause. In fact, some women actually find that any testosterone they do have converts to estrogen in perimenopause. (Estrogen blocker supplements like DIM and calcium d-glucarate can help. See Chapter 6 for more information.)

Preserving Testosterone

As you approach perimenopause, it's important to be proactive and take steps to maintain your testosterone levels. An important thing you can do is lower your consumption of alcohol or stop drinking alcohol altogether. As I'm writing this, I know this particular piece of advice will not be received well. Drinking is a popular pastime, I get it! With that said, drinking too much is associated with decreased testosterone levels and the price you pay for that can be so high that it may make it worthwhile to drink less or stop drinking altogether for periods of time.

Specific ways that alcohol affects testosterone levels include:[51]

- When we drink alcohol, NAD+, which is a coenzyme that synthesizes testosterone, must help with alcohol metabolism instead.

- Drinking alcohol releases certain endorphins that can interfere with testosterone synthesis.

- Alcohol can increase a stress hormone called cortisol, which is known to decrease testosterone synthesis.

- Alcohol may increase the conversion of testosterone to estrogen in the body.

Let me be clear: I'm not telling anyone to stop drinking alcohol, but if you are in perimenopause you are at risk of low testosterone levels and even moderate alcohol use will make things worse.

Alcohol Use in Women Is Increasing

I grappled with whether to include an entire section of this guide on alcohol, but ultimately I decided to for several reasons.

- Several women with whom I spoke as I wrote this guide shared that, for them, perimenopause coincided with shifts in their lives that led to greater alcohol use. For example, they have older children who require less day-to-day hands-on caregiving, giving them more free time to

---

51   www.healthline.com/health/how-alcohol-affects-testosterone#effect-on-testosterone

indulge. They also have more disposable income than they did ten or fifteen years ago so don't feel badly spending money on alcohol.

- More women are drinking in midlife, period. A new study shows binge drinking is happening more among middle-aged women.[52] According to the study, the male-to-female gender gap has been narrowing over the past century and binge drinking and alcohol use disorder (AUD) are increasing more rapidly in women in age groups forty-five to sixty-four and sixty-five and older. The study authors don't know exactly why this increase in high-risk drinking is occurring, but they offer numerous potential reasons, including:

- Stress from work.

- Stress from retirement.

- Financial pressures.

- Empty nest.

- Challenges associated with menopause (I would add perimenopause to this!).

In the past decade the alcohol industry has turned its attention and marketing dollars toward women big time! It's "pink-washing" alcohol by creating marketing campaigns that highlight alcohol with other products such as makeup, promoting "low calorie" alcohol as better for women and even associating drinking with gender

---

52   www.contemporaryobgyn.net/view/older-women-are-consuming-more-alcohol

empowerment. Nothing ticks me off more than being manipulated, especially when women's health is at risk. And it is. Our hormones are our health!

Numerous other studies have shown that many, many women drink alcohol as a way to cope with stress, trauma or other challenges.[53] As you've read in this guide, perimenopause can be very destabilizing and many of us lack the support we need. It's not surprising that some women may be turning to alcohol as a way to manage this stage of life.

I'll also mention that there are greater problems with increased alcohol use beyond the fact that it affects our hormone levels. Women can become addicted to alcohol with less exposure over shorter periods of time because we don't metabolize alcohol quickly. Perhaps scariest of all: according to the National Cancer Institute, alcohol is a carcinogen.[54] We just don't need those worries on top of dealing with perimenopause itself. Again, my goal here is not to get on a soapbox about alcohol. My hope, though, is that I've given you a better sense of how alcohol affects our hormones as well as how it may affect our health overall.

53   Peltier, MacKenzie R et al. "Sex differences in stress-related alcohol use." *Neurobiology of stress* vol. 10 100149. 8 Feb. 2019, doi:10.1016/j.ynstr.2019.100149

54   www.cancer.gov/about-cancer/causes-prevention/risk/alcohol/alcohol-fact-sheet

Chapter 11:

SLEEPING BEAUTY STRATEGIES

> **"THE DAY I HIT FORTY-ONE, IT WAS LIKE MY** body decided it could no longer sleep through the night. I woke up at 2:30 a.m. for five straight years, anxiously rolling around in bed hoping I could fall back to sleep. I did fall back to sleep about 40 percent of the time, but the cumulative effect of not getting sound sleep for all those years really took a toll on me. It was worse than when my kids were little, worse than when we adopted two puppies at the same time. I never want to experience that again." — Pam

There is nothing I love more than a good night's sleep. I know I'm not the only one! As much as I love sleep, I've been plagued my whole life with a curse: I need tons of sleep, but I'm also the lightest sleeper so everything and anything disrupts my sleep. Enter perimenopause and things went downhill fast. I was already exhausted from undiagnosed thyroid disease when I began to find it harder and harder to fall asleep and stay asleep. I am not alone in that struggle. It turns out that perimenopause hormone imbalance is the culprit. Hormones are "chemical messengers" that regulate bodily functions like sleep and as those hormones shift, regulation issues arise. Keep in mind that sleep is incredibly important to our health and well-being.[55] Our bodies need sleep and do not do well without it. Here are some hormones that play a part in our perimenopausal sleep challenges.

Melatonin is a hormone released into our bloodstream to promote a regular sleep-wake cycle. As we age, our bodies release less and less melatonin, which results in disturbances to our sleep-wake cycle.

Progesterone is the "calming" and sleep-promoting hormone. Progesterone increases production of GABA, a neurotransmitter that helps us sleep. Low progesterone causes anxiety, restlessness and trouble sleeping, including waking up frequently during the night.

Estrogen (and estradiol, which is a form of estrogen) promotes healthy sleep by helping the body use serotonin and other neurochemicals that assist sleep. Balanced estrogen levels contribute to higher-quality sleep, with fewer awakenings throughout the night and less time needed to fall asleep.

Follicle-stimulating hormone (FSH) plays a key role in our menstrual cycles. As FSH levels rise, the quality of our sleep worsens. Prior to perimenopause, FSH causes ovarian follicles to enlarge and produce estrogen, which in turn shuts off the FSH production. When we are in perimenopause there are fewer ovarian follicles to be stimulated and our estrogen levels decline. This decline in estrogen leads to an increase in FSH because there isn't enough estrogen being produced to turn off our body's production of FSH.

---

55 Worley, Susan L. "The Extraordinary Importance of Sleep: The Detrimental Effects of Inadequate Sleep on Health and Public Safety Drive an Explosion of Sleep Research." *P & T: A peer-reviewed journal for formulary management* vol. 43,12 (2018): 758–763.

If you are in perimenopause and experiencing insomnia and sleep issues, you are not alone. In fact, according to a 2017 Centers for Disease Control (CDC) survey, sleep problems tend to increase significantly during perimenopause:[56]

- More than half of perimenopausal women—56 percent—sleep less than seven hours a night on average.

- Nearly one-quarter—24.8 percent—of perimenopausal women say they have trouble falling asleep four or more times in a week.

- Even more common than trouble falling asleep? Difficulty staying asleep. Among women in perimenopause, 30.8 percent say they have trouble staying asleep at least four nights a week.

- Half of perimenopausal women—49.9 percent—wake in the morning feeling tired, rather than rested, four or more days in a week.

- Twenty-six percent of women experience severe symptoms that impact daytime functioning and qualify them for a diagnosis of insomnia.[57]

Is it just me or is this totally unacceptable?!! Half of perimenopausal women wake in the morning feeling tired four or more days in a week?!! How are we supposed to excel in our careers, care for children and older family members, interact healthfully with our intimate

---

56   www.cdc.gov/nchs/products/databriefs/db286.htm

57   Baker, Fiona C et al. "Sleep problems during the menopausal transition: Prevalence, impact, and management challenges." *Nature and science of sleep* vol. 10 73–95. 9 Feb. 2018, doi:10.2147/NSS.S125807

partners and more on no sleep? I know women are awesome, but I feel like this is asking too much of us. Here's the irony: healthy amounts of sleep are necessary to balance our hormones. When we don't get enough sleep our cortisol and our glucose levels rise. Over time these changes can affect our thyroid and sex hormones. A vicious cycle!

Unfortunately, I did not receive a lot of support in the early days of perimenopause. I remember asking a doctor what I should do about my insomnia, and she said: "It's perimenopause, it happens." And that was that as far as she was concerned. Unless you do your homework now, you could find yourself in the same boat. Prepare now! Here are the specific steps I recommend you take before and during perimenopause to get the amount of sleep you need and deserve:

1. Test your hormones! By now, you had to know I was going to say that.

2. Find a clinician who specializes in hormone balancing.

3. Track your sleep.

4. Look into herbal remedies.

5. Adopt good sleep strategies and be vigilant about them.

6. Advocate for yourself.

7. Reduce stress (yes, I know this is easier said than done).

Let's break each of these recommendations down into detail.

TEST YOUR HORMONES AND FIND THE RIGHT CLINICIAN

As always, first and foremost, you need to know where your hormone levels are to understand whether and how hormones may be affecting your sleep. If you are a couple of years into perimenopause, there's a very good chance your progesterone has tanked. If you are getting closer to menopause, it means your estrogen levels are lower than they've ever been. As you read on the previous page, your progesterone and estrogen levels affect sleep, so it's important to test your hormones to get a sense of where you stand. If you are early in perimenopause and working with a clinician who specializes in hormone balancing, they will likely give you a prescription for progesterone. Progesterone was a game changer for me when it came to sleep, and many women have had similar experiences. Clinicians who work with perimenopausal women regularly will put the puzzle pieces together quickly and help you get back to a healthy sleep cycle.

TRACK YOUR SLEEP

An effective clinician will want to know exactly what kinds of sleep issues you are experiencing. Sleep issues are not one size fits all, and the solutions to address sleep issues are not either. Set aside a two-week period and track the following:

- Time you get into bed.

- About long it takes to fall asleep. This does not have to be exact.

- How often you wake and how long you stay awake during those times. Again, this does not have to be exact, especially if looking at a clock keeps you awake longer.

- What time you get out of bed.

Share this information with your care team after you've gathered at least two weeks of data about your sleep.

LOOK INTO HERBAL REMEDIES

Before I knew I was in perimenopause and before I discovered the magic of progesterone, I did a lot of research into herbal remedies for sleep. I was scared of things like Ambien and other prescription medications, so I tested lots of different options, including all of the remedies listed next. I can vouch for **Valerian, Passionflower and Cannabidiol (CBD)**. I still use **Soul CBD Dream Gummies** right before my period each month, which is when my sleep cycle tends to get screwed up even though I take oral progesterone nightly without fail.

Keep in mind that while I am sharing with you the research I did and the various herbal options I tested, you must do your own due diligence as I am not a medical professional or an herbalist. Do your own research to determine which of these medicines might work best for you and how much of them to take if you do decide to use them to help with sleep. Work with your care team or an herbalist to make these decisions. If you choose to take any of these remedies, please be transparent with your health-care providers in order to avoid any dangerous medication combinations or issues.

Cannabidiol (CBD). Cannabidiol—also known as CBD—is one of the main cannabinoids in the cannabis plant. Cannabinoids interact with our endocannabinoid system, which helps our bodies maintain a state of balance. Cannabidiol does not contain THC, which is what makes people "high" when they use marijuana. A 2017 review looked at multiple studies on the safety of CBD and concluded it's a relatively safe treatment to help with anxiety and to ensure more REM sleep.[58] I

---

58   Iffland, Kerstin, and Franjo Grotenhermen. "An Update on Safety and Side Effects of Cannabidiol: A Review of Clinical Data and Relevant Animal Studies." *Cannabis and cannabinoid research* vol. 2,1 139–154. 1 Jun. 2017, doi:10.1089/can.2016.0034

have **used Royal CBD** successfully and buy it via their website: https://royalcbd.com. I have also had great success with **Soul CBD Dream Gummies**, which have passionflower, magnesium and melatonin as well as CBD. I consider them the "big guns" and only take them a couple of times a month when my sleep is really off due to my impending monthly period. They can be bought via the **Soul CBD** website: www.mysoulcbd.com/products/dream-cbd-capsules.

> **IMPORTANT NOTE:** CBD is **not monitored by the Food and Drug Administration the same way medications are.** You can't always be certain of what you're getting and whether it's safe. CBD contents may not be consistent and may include other ingredients. Remember, natural doesn't always mean safe. Proceed with caution and do your own research.

Korean Red Ginseng. Ginseng is a short, slow-growing plant with fleshy roots. There are two types of ginseng: American and Asian. The roots of Korean red ginseng have been tested and shown to help with sleep disturbances, including insomnia.[59] Similar to melatonin, it is recommended that Korean red ginseng only be used for short-term sleep issues.

Melatonin. Melatonin is a natural hormone that plays a role in our sleep-wake cycle. It is synthesized mainly by the pineal gland located in the brain. Melatonin supplements are widely used to help people fall asleep and stay asleep; however, it is recommended that melatonin only be used for short-term sleep issues.

---

59   Lee, Chung-Il et al. "Repeated Administration of Korea Red Ginseng Extract Increases Non-rapid Eye Movement Sleep via GABAAergic Systems." *Journal of ginseng research* vol. 36,4 (2012): 403–410. doi:10.5142/jgr.2012.36.4.403

Passionflower. Passionflower is a climbing vine with white and purple flowers. Passionflower is native to the southeastern United States and Central and South America. The chemicals in passionflower have calming effects, so many people use passionflower to ease anxiety and for insomnia. Studies on passionflower have found it to be effective for sleep. I have used the **Now** brand successfully.[60]

Valerian. Valerian is a tall, flowering grassland plant. The extract of the root of valerian has been widely used to treat sleeping disorders in countries around the world for decades because valerian seems to act like a sedative on the brain and nervous system. I found it helped with my anxiety and allowed me to relax enough to fall asleep. I have used the **Nature's Bounty** brand successfully.

> **IMPORTANT NOTE: Herbal supplements are not monitored by the FDA the same way medications are.** You can't always be certain of what you're getting and whether it's safe. Herbal supplement contents may not be consistent and may include other ingredients. Remember, natural doesn't always mean safe. When selecting a brand of supplements, look for products that have been third party tested and contain safe levels of vitamins and minerals.

USE GOOD SLEEP STRATEGIES

Many of us are our own worst enemies when it comes to sleep. We know a good night's sleep is important, but we don't make sleep a

---

60   Donath F, Quispe S, Diefenbach K, Maurer A, Fietze I, Roots I. Critical evaluation of the effect of valerian extract on sleep structure and sleep quality. Pharmacopsychiatry. 2000 Mar;33(2):47–53. doi: 10.1055/s-2000-7972. PMID: 10761819.

priority. Why? Here are some of the things I do that prevent me from getting enough sleep:

- I catch up on all of the things I'm behind on at night. I say to myself, "I'm just going to get a couple more things done before tomorrow," and when I look at the clock four hours later, it's 1:00 a.m.

- I binge watch Netflix. I don't have a ton of vices, but Netflix is definitely one of them. Recently I've started to realize that even though I'm usually lying down when I watch Netflix, television actually stimulates me, so much so that I have a hard time falling asleep.

- I surf Instagram in order to plan vacations. Scroll, scroll, scroll—crap; it's midnight!

I know I can't be the only one who does these things. I wish I knew five years ago how much good sleep affects my mood and hormones because I would have started adopting better habits back then. With that said, it's never too late to reset a priority. Here are six things I have started doing to get a better night's sleep:

1. I plug my phone in downstairs three or four nights a week at 9:00 p.m. and I don't look at it until the morning. Notice I'm only up to three or four nights a week of doing this. That's because I'm not perfect and it's okay. Progress, not perfection, is my goal.

2. I bought **SleepBuds II from Bose**. You can find them on the Bose website. They're incredibly comfortable to wear as a side sleeper and the white noise helps a light sleeper like me conk me out quickly and helps me fall back to sleep quickly if I wake

up for any reason. And yes, they're an investment, but they have changed my life.

3. I've created a new bedtime routine: lights out by 10:00 p.m.—no exceptions—and no television after 9:00 p.m. It's clear to me that my body needs an hour of quiet stretching, reading, journaling etc. to "come down off the day," so I build that in and by the time 10:00 p.m. rolls around I can barely keep my eyes open. In the winter I move my bedtime to 9:30 p.m. because I can tell my body wants to take advantage of the extra darkness and hibernate.

4. I stop working on my to-do list by 8:00 p.m. My brain is pretty tired by 8:00 p.m. anyway, so I've decided to stop pushing myself to catch up on things in the evenings. Bonus: I've found that going to bed earlier and getting a good night sleep means I'm not dragging during the day, so I have an easier time getting stuff done.

5. I go to bed at the same time as many nights as possible. This is the most challenging change I made to my routine in perimenopause. I've always been good about going to bed fairly early during the week, but I allowed myself to stay up late and sleep in on the weekends. I didn't realize I was confusing my body and it was always trying to catch up. As lame as it may sound, it's a rare Friday or Saturday evening when I'm awake past 10:00 p.m., but it has been life-changing. Whereas I was exhausted for the first five to eight years of perimenopause, I now feel well rested most days.

6. I get sunlight on my face in the morning whenever possible. It turns out our eyes need light to help set our internal clock.

Early morning sunlight in particular seems to help us get to sleep at night. As we age, our eyes are less able to take in light, which means we become more likely to have problems going to sleep. The easiest way for me to get sunlight in the morning is by walking one of the many dogs I have. When that isn't an option because I have an early work call or the weather is not ideal, I use a sunlight lamp, which I keep on my desk year round, and it produces the same effects. I use a **Carex** lamp.

I want to acknowledge two things about these changes I made to prioritize more and better sleep:

- I recognize establishing a new sleep routine can be a challenge. It's a life change and requires commitment. One way to make it a little more palatable is to adopt one change at a time and take your time. Progress, not perfection!

- This is my schedule, and it is based the fact that I'm an early bird. You may be a night owl or have different habits you want to work on. What matters is consistency and getting a full and restful night of sleep on a regular basis.

Advocate for Yourself

When it comes to getting the sleep you need and deserve in perimenopause, I highly recommend advocating for yourself. Friends, colleagues, family and even your care team may diminish any sleep challenges you experience, but I'm here to tell you: sleep is important! If your care team doesn't take your sleep concerns seriously, find a new care team. If you are open to hormone replacement, ask your doctor if a prescription for progesterone or estrogen is right for you. So many of us have become sleep deprived over the course of many years that we may not even remember what a good night's sleep feels like or the last time we got one. As "normal" as that may appear, it's actually not. Adequate sleep is key to our health and well-being and to keeping our hormones in balance.

Reduce Stress

The final recommendation I have related to getting adequate sleep in perimenopause is to reduce stress. I won't go into this in great detail in this section because the next chapter provides lots of advice and guidance, but the bottom line is this: stress directly impacts our sleep quality and chronic stress often leads to insomnia. If you are not yet in perimenopause begin now to think of the ways you can reduce or eliminate stress in your life. A life with less stress will help you significantly when you are in perimenopause and dealing with hormone shifts. I know this is easier said than done, so I share some tips and recommendations in upcoming sections. Keep reading!

Chapter 12:

MOVING OUR BODIES

> **"ONE OF THE SURVIVAL STRATEGIES I USED**
> in perimenopause was movement. Moving my body was a game
> changer for me. It centered my mind and calmed my emotions. But
> I had to adopt a new mindset when it came to exercise. Instead
> of focusing on looking good, which I had been doing my whole
> life, I looked at exercise as a way to care for my body as it went
> through some serious hormonal shifts." — *Siobhan*

As I've written many times in this guide so far, being *prepared* for perimenopause is ideal. Exercise is one of the ways to manage perimenopause symptoms, so if you are not exercising now, my hope is that this section will encourage you to do so. Establishing an exercise routine now will mean you will have established a habit by the time you enter perimenopause. If you exercise currently on a regular basis, this section will help you think about the most effective ways to move your body during the perimenopause stage. If you're already in perimenopause, I think this section will still be helpful to you. Read on!

When I entered perimenopause, I was dealing with a new thyroid diagnosis and had gained nineteen pounds. I could barely keep my eyes open from sleepless nights due to plummeting progesterone levels. Every fiber of my body ached from lack of testosterone. On top of that, I was mentally beating myself up daily. I blamed my rapid weight gain on not exercising enough (or the right way) instead of my underactive thyroid. I couldn't figure out what I was doing wrong. I had been pushing myself for years—lots and lots of exercise and eating well—so I'm not sure why I was blaming myself, but I did. I adopted the mindset of if what I'm doing isn't working, I must do it more.

Please, please, please, don't do this to yourself! If what you're doing isn't working, your body is trying to tell you something. And, if you're in perimenopause, hormones, including your thyroid, are likely the culprit. I pushed my body so hard I eventually hit the wall. I remember sitting on the couch in my living room sobbing my eyes out. I had never felt so exhausted in my entire life, including caring for newborns. Any kind of physical activity sidelined me for days. I secretly thought I had a deadly disease. At one point, my husband turned to me and said, "I'm really worried about you," and that's when I knew I needed to take a new path.

My new path involved treating my hormones while also stepping away from all physical activity except walking for about six months. That break from my typical, somewhat grueling workout regimen, along with the appropriate dose of thyroid medicine and testosterone replacement therapy, finally gave my body a chance to heal. Let me be clear: those six months were *hard*. I missed my exercise routines and I worried not exercising would result in more weight gain. (That didn't happen, by the way. In fact, I lost weight due to finally having a working thyroid again.) But that break was critical for me. If you have significant physical symptoms related to perimenopause or thyroid disease, you can't pretend that your body will continue to work as it once did. An adjustment period, whatever that looks like for you, is absolutely necessary.

WHY EXERCISE?

Here's the thing, we've all heard "eat right and exercise" our whole lives. You'd have to be living under a rock not to know exercise is good for our bodies. With that said, if you are able and not dealing with significant perimenopause or thyroid disease symptoms, exercise is particularly important during perimenopause for the following reasons:

- We lose muscle mass as we age and muscle is the engine of our metabolism. Muscle also keeps us strong, which is important as we age.

- When a woman enters the perimenopausal state, natural testosterone production (critical to muscles, bones and protein synthesis) can decrease by more than 50 percent and exercise can help increase or maintain testosterone levels.

- Our bones become more brittle in our forties and fifties. Weight lifting can strengthen them.

- We lose flexibility as we age.

- Exercise can help decrease some of the physical and emotional symptoms of perimenopause.

- Dehydration brought on by perimenopause can lead to constipation whereas exercise keeps things moving.

When you look at exercise broadly, you can see exercise has additional benefits that have absolutely nothing to do with perimenopause, but are certainly worth mentioning: exercise increases longevity, meaning exercisers live longer on the whole, and regular exercise decreases the risk of cardiorespiratory and metabolic diseases and some cancers (most notably colon and breast).[61]

EXERCISES TO PRIORITIZE

How can exercise help us in perimenopause and what kinds of exercise should we prioritize? Here are my recommendations and what I have found helpful (with some research data to back me up!):

Weight Lifting. Weight lifting is the number one exercise to prioritize in perimenopause. It builds muscle, reduces fat, strengthens our bones and helps our bodies produce testosterone naturally. There's a lot of back and forth in the fitness world about whether people should "lift heavy" weights for fewer repetitions or lift lighter weights for lots of repetitions. I'm not going to wade into the debate because the most important message I want to convey is *lift weights, any weights, consistently*. That's my bottom line. If you are not yet in perimenopause, begin lifting weights now.

Having a weight-lifting routine going into perimenopause will help reduce the muscle loss that comes with perimenopause. If you are already in perimenopause, begin lifting today. Our risk of osteoporosis skyrockets once we're in menopause, so get into a routine pronto.

I've done both heavy and light lifting and both have worked well for me. I've seen my muscle mass increase, the "flab" decrease and I find that I release endorphins while lifting weights. This is so great because

---

61 Sternfeld, Barbara, and Sheila Dugan. "Physical activity and health during the menopausal transition." *Obstetrics and gynecology clinics of North America* vol. 38,3 (2011): 537–566. doi:10.1016/j.ogc.2011.05.008

our moods can be a challenge in perimenopause. Even on the hardest days, I feel a "high" after lifting weights that can't be beat.

I know some women reading this are thinking: "I don't have time for one more thing in my life, let alone bench pressing!" I get it, I really do. Here's the thing: you don't need to go to the gym. I have a set of weights next to my desk, a bunch of fitness bands in my office and in my kitchen and a set of weights next to the TV in the bedroom. Whenever I'm on a conference call, I pick up a weight or a band and whenever I put a television show on, I do some repetitions. Yes, I'm particularly enthusiastic!

The other nice thing about lifting weights is you can often "see" the results of your efforts more quickly than other types of exercise. My mother is in her late seventies and started using weights during her water aerobics class and I could totally see her new muscles after only six weeks! Not only that, she is walking more erect than she has in years.

People have told me they have no idea where to start when it comes to weight lifting. The Internet is your friend. Go to Fitness Blender or YouTube or Instagram and you'll find millions of weight-lifting programs and exercises to try. Women have also shared with me that they find weight lifting boring. I'm not sure what to say except do you remember the saying: "Only brush the teeth you want to keep"? Lifting is the same thing: "Only lift the muscles you want to keep." If weight lifting sounds awful, do it while you're distracted by other things: watch a movie, listen to an audio book etc.

Mobility Exercises. Mobility exercises are the second type of exercise I suggest prioritizing before and during perimenopause as well as into menopause and beyond. This is a broad category into which I include the following: Yoga, Pilates, Tai Chi, stretching, balance work,

Barre and body specific exercises like hip stabilization. My hope is that you, my dear reader, are younger than me (age forty-nine) because, boy, oh boy, do I wish I had devoted more time to this category in my late thirties and early-to-mid forties. Unfortunately, I was addicted to cardiovascular exercise. It's not too late for you! It's also not too late for me, and I've leaned in hard to these types of exercise in recent years.

Mobility exercises are important because as we age our bodies become less flexible, we lose our sense of balance, our joints stop cooperating and our bones become more brittle. Add to this the fact that so many of us spend our days sitting down at desks all day everyday (as I type this I've been seated for at least two hours: argh!!) and it's not surprising that we tend to have mobility issues as we get older. Do me a favor and type "sit to stand test" into your favorite Internet search application. This is the test that will assess our physical functionality if we're lucky enough to get to our seventies. It may look easy to you today, but give yourself twenty-five years of not working on balance and mobility and it will feel impossible!

I highly recommend getting creative and adventurous. For example, try Tai Chi, which can have a positive impact on your bone health.[62] Go to a relaxing Yoga class, which can be very soothing and offset some of the anxiety many of us experience in perimenopause.[63] However, like most things in life, we tend to be consistent when we

---

62　Sun Z, Chen H, Berger MR, Zhang L, Guo H, Huang Y. Effects of tai chi exercise on bone health in perimenopausal and postmenopausal women: A systematic review and meta analysis. Osteoporos Int. 2016 Oct;27(10):2901–2911. doi: 10.1007/s00198-016-3626-3. Epub 2016 May 23. PMID: 27216996.

63　Naomi M. Simon, Stefan G. Hofmann, David Rosenfield et al. **Efficacy of Yoga vs. Cognitive Behavioral Therapy vs. Stress Education for the Treatment of Generalized Anxiety Disorder: A Randomized Clinical Trial.** *JAMA Psychiatry*, 2020 DOI: 10.1001/jamapsychiatry.2020.2496

enjoy what we're doing or we can readily see the benefits of our efforts. So if you hate Yoga, don't do it! If you're like most people and short on time, look for "two-fers" wherever you can. For example, I add in balance exercises when I lift. Experiment a bit to see what works for you.

A couple of years ago I committed to doing Pilates three times a week for a year. I was like a dog with a bone dutifully following through with my commitment, and I can truly say my abs and back have never been stronger. But, when the year was up, I was over Pilates. This was about three years ago and I haven't done a class since and that's okay. It will still be there for me if I ever decide to get back into it.

Cardiovascular. Cardiovascular exercise is the third type of I exercise I recommend for women in perimenopause. While I believe cardio exercise is important, again, my personal recommendation is to prioritize weight lifting and mobility exercises over cardio. I do also recommend cardio exercise for the following reasons:

1. When we move our bodies enough to sweat, we stimulate our lymphatic systems, which are responsible for moving toxins out of our bodies. This is especially important if you are estrogen dominant.

2. When we do cardio exercise at a high enough rate, our bodies release endorphins, the "feel good" hormones that relieve the anxiety and depression many of us experience in perimenopause.

3. Cardio is good for our hearts. As we age, we are more susceptible to strokes and heart attacks and cardio exercise can lower our risk for these conditions. It can also increase the likelihood of surviving a heart attack should you have one.

Here's the most important thing to remember when it comes to cardio: don't limit yourself! One of the women I interviewed for the book shared with me that she stopped doing cardio when she became too tired to run. She felt like anything less than a five-mile run wasn't good enough. If you can't run anymore, walk! If you love dancing, dance! If the Stairmaster or bike are your favorite machines, use those. Just move your body!

Let me say a little bit more about walking: at the beginning of this chapter I mentioned I gave up all exercise except walking for six months. Let me tell you, walking is like a miracle drug! I used walks during that time to decompress from work, to give my brain a break, to be in and enjoy nature and to listen to music, which always brings me joy. No matter what was happening in my life, I always came back from those walks "lighter" emotionally and some of my best ideas—whether personal or work-related—came to me on those walks. I realize not everyone has access to safe walking areas and I consider myself fortunate. If safety is an issue, walking indoors also works. You don't need a treadmill or fancy equipment. Walk the perimeter of a room while listening to music.

EXERCISE COMBINING

Here's the tricky thing I've learned with exercise: we need to combine these three types of exercise in perimenopause in order to get the best results. For example, walking four days a week is great for our mental health and it stimulates our lymphatic system, but it doesn't stave off muscle loss. Additionally, too much cardio exercise in particular can lead to overuse injuries. Here is what I recommend:

Weight lifting. At least two days a week, ideally three. Remember, you don't have to spend hours in the gym; just lift heavy things a couple of times a week. I lift for thirty minutes twice a week and it does the trick.

Mobility exercise. Ideally, a couple of minutes daily but a least four days a week. I probably lost a lot of you just now. Sorry! I'm pretty hard-core about this because I've struggled with body pain and injuries from not investing enough time in mobility exercises. The challenge is that body pain and injuries end up making all kinds of exercise more difficult, meaning you do less of it, which can exacerbate perimenopause symptoms. Try and commit to something small every day: ten minutes of Yoga, fifteen minutes of dynamic stretching, five minutes of balancing. You and your joints will thank me in your fifties!

Cardio. Three days a week maximum and ideally forty to fifty minutes maximum at a time. This has been the toughest perimenopause habit for me to adopt. I love tennis and I love hiking. I hiked three miles every day with my dogs for at least six years. I was definitely a big fan of cardio. Unfortunately, it broke down my body and did nothing to help with muscle loss. Don't go there! I now do cardio three days a week at the most. I do it to get my heart rate up to protect myself from heart disease, I do it for fun, and I do it because my body tends to hold onto toxins easily and sweating with cardio exercise helps release them. It can help you in these ways too. This is not to say that I don't move my body throughout the day. I have lots of dogs who need walks (versus hikes) so I sprinkle those in throughout my day. I walk to errands whenever I can, and I often will take a stroll in my neighborhood in the evenings. I'm sure you can think of ways to keep active that you can slip into your life and lifestyle too!

IMPORTANT NOTE: If your body is in pain more often than not, if you are struggling to get through your day because you're exhausted all of the time, or if you have experienced rapid weight gain, exercise should not be your priority. Getting to the bottom of those symptoms is the most important thing you can do.

SOME FINAL THOUGHTS

If you look closely at this chapter, you will notice I have included nothing about exercise and its effects on weight. That's because for the vast majority of people, weight has much more to do with the food and drinks we consume, not whether or how we move our bodies. It's also because while weight can be an issue for many of us in perimenopause, it is likely due to hormones being out of balance more than anything else.

I also do not want to in any way add to the chorus of voices that tell us to exercise to be thin or to look a certain way. The message I hope you'll take away from this chapter is that exercise is critical for our health and well-being—healthy hearts, joints etc.—and can help us manage our hormones. I want to acknowledge that exercise is not an enjoyable activity for many people. I hope this chapter hasn't been too much of a downer for you.

Chapter 13:

MONITOR MENTAL HEALTH

> **"THE HARDEST PART OF PERIMENOPAUSE** for me has been that my mental health has hit rock bottom. I'm anxious all of the time and I'm struggling with depression again. I feel like I'm constantly on edge for no reason. Everything frustrates me and I don't feel like myself anymore" — *Melanie*

Before writing this guide, I spoke with and interviewed many, many women. Some were beyond perimenopause and told me the changes to their mental health were the biggest challenge they faced in this stage of life. Many other women I spoke with were not yet in perimenopause, and the majority of those women told me their biggest perimenopause worry is that their mental and emotional health will suffer.

It broke my heart every time a woman shared with me how fearful she is for her mental well-being and how little support she felt she had at her disposal to navigate perimenopause. Ladies, this just isn't cool! We need and deserve to know how our mental health may be affected in perimenopause so we can prepare ourselves and come up with an effective game plan. My hope is that this section will give you some valuable information and a roadmap for action.

MENTAL HEALTH AWARENESS HAS IMPROVED IN RECENT DECADES

In many ways, we've come a long way when it comes to mental health. I was born in the 1970s and my comfort level and experience with mental health is light-years ahead of my parents and their peers. It feels like many more people in my generation are tapped into our emotional and mental health, whereas many of our parents were taught to ignore their feelings and certainly not to show them. Lots of women my age have benefited from talk therapy. Many of us have also learned strategies to manage our stress. Others of us have greatly benefited from medicines that help our bodies produce chemicals we don't naturally create.

MENTAL HEALTH ISSUES ARE ON THE RISE AND WOMEN ARE MORE SUSCEPTIBLE

Despite the progress made in the past three decades, mental health issues like anxiety and depression are on the rise. People are struggling. In addition, in my experience a deep stigma remains firmly in place when it comes to mental and emotional health challenges. This is the case despite these staggering statistics:

- According to the World Health Organization, one in four people in the world will be affected by mental or neurological disorders at some point in their lives. Around 450 million people currently suffer from such conditions, placing mental disorders among the leading causes of ill health and disability worldwide.

- Numbers like this are difficult to read because they underscore the degree to which mental health issues affect us as a humanity. What's worse is that the World Health Organization found that between 30 and 80 percent of people with mental health issues don't seek treatment. In my experience, many of us delay treatment or avoid seeking treatment because of the stigma I mentioned. We fear being treated differently by friends, family, coworkers and society in general.

Add to all of this a very important statistic to keep in mind as you prepare for perimenopause: *Women are twice as likely as men to suffer from depressive symptoms and disorder.*[64]

Read that again. Twice as likely.

PERIMENOPAUSE CAN AFFECT MENTAL AND EMOTIONAL HEALTH

Here's the thing: context matters. Just by virtue of being women, we are twice as likely as men to experience depression. Additionally, by the time we get to perimenopause most of us will have lived more than thirty-five years on the planet. The vast majority of us will have experienced challenging and traumatic things that affect our mental well-being. We likely are aware of and have experienced personally the powerful stigma that makes talking about or receiving support for our mental and emotional well-being a challenge. My requests:

---

64 Bromberger, Joyce T, and Howard M Kravitz. "Mood and menopause: Findings from the Study of Women's Health across the Nation (SWAN) over 10 years." *Obstetrics and gynecology clinics of North America* vol. 38,3 (2011): 609–625. doi:10.1016/j.ogc.2011.05.011

- Pay attention to your mental health in perimenopause. I know many of us put our needs last after our families, our careers etc., but we need to take care of ourselves. Ignoring your mental health doesn't do anyone any favors. In fact, ignoring our own needs has the potential to endanger our health, relationships, careers and more. Perimenopause can be a challenging time with changes to our bodies and to our mental health. Perimenopause is not a time to put your needs on the back burner. It's a time to be on the lookout for changes in your moods.

- If you are struggling, seek out help. I know from personal experience it's hard to ask for help, but please fight the urge to "power through." And, let go of any shame you may feel because I'm here to tell you there is nothing to be embarrassed about. Go back and read the statistics on the previous page. Many, many people struggle with mental and emotional health issues. They are not character flaws: they are *health* issues.

This next part is VERY IMPORTANT! I apologize for the all caps, but I know how busy everyone is and there's a chance that you're skimming this guide. I don't want you to miss this part, so read the next section very closely. When it comes to perimenopause and mental and emotional well-being, it's important to keep in mind that your history matters. *Women with a history of depression, anxiety, bipolar or other mental or emotional health conditions are at greater risk of experiencing depression or exacerbated bipolar symptoms during perimenopause.*[65]

---

65 www.npr.org/sections/health-shots/2020/01/16/796682276/
for-some-women-nearing-menopause-depression-and-anxiety-can-spike

I was completely unaware of this fact to prior to writing this guide. Here's the frustrating thing: I experienced postpartum depression after my first child was born. Despite this, not one medical professional cautioned me when I was in my late thirties or at any time during my forties that I was at greater risk of experiencing depression in perimenopause. When I was pregnant with my second child, I was impressed with how diligent my first child's pediatrician and my OB/GYN were about asking me at every check-up how my moods were and if I were in danger of harming myself or my child. They prescribed an antidepressant during the final weeks of my pregnancy and continued to check on me post-partum.

Why is it that none of the health professionals (e.g., my OB-GYN, primary care doctor) I encountered in my thirties and forties inquired about my past mental and emotional health or shared the important information about risk with me? Perhaps it's because, as I mentioned in the early part of this guide, most doctors receive less than one hour of training on women's health issues after their reproductive years. Essentially, if you've made it this far in the guide, you're almost as knowledgeable about perimenopause as a lot of health-care professionals.

PREPARE NOW IF YOU HAVE EXPERIENCED MENTAL AND EMOTIONAL HEALTH CHALLENGES

Knowledge is power. If you have experienced anxiety, depression, bipolar disorder etc. at any time in your life, you need to prepare now for perimenopause. I recommend the following steps:

1. If you are experiencing depression or are suicidal right now, go to your nearest emergency department or call 911 immediately.

2. Track your moods, your feelings and any signs of depression, anxiety, or other mental or emotional health conditions. Go to www.helloperiwinkle.com/tracker to download our Well-Being Tracker.

3. Confide in a trusted friend or family member. Let them know you are approaching perimenopause or are in perimenopause and share the statistics from this guide. Ask them to be on the lookout for any changes in your moods or behavior and encourage them to speak with you if they observe anything. If you are worried you might be resistant to feedback from a family member or friend, come up with a code word so your family member or friend doesn't have to go into great detail about what they're observing. For example, they could just say or text "pink bunny" and that would be a sign to you that you are showing signs of a mental health crisis.

4. Work with both a mental health-care professional and a health-care provider with expertise in women's health, specifically hormone balancing, *now*. Make an appointment to see them. Tell them both your history and ask them what you should know and do to protect against experiencing mental and emotional issues in perimenopause. Connect them to each other so they are both aware of any treatment or medications you are taking.

While this information comes too late for me, and perhaps even for some of you reading this guide, here's some good news: in 2018 NAMS and the Women and Mood Disorders Task Force of the National Network of Depression Centers released the first-ever guidelines for the evaluation and treatment of perimenopausal depression. These guidelines have also been endorsed by the International Menopause

Society. These guidelines represent huge progress because when guidelines are available for a condition, it means the condition is recognized. My hope is that all health-care providers who focus on hormone balancing will adopt these guidelines and ensure mental health treatment is incorporated into perimenopause and menopause care.

WHAT IF YOU HAVE NO HISTORY OF MENTAL OR EMOTIONAL CONDITIONS?

Even if you do not have a history of depression or other mental or emotional conditions you still may experience mental or emotional changes during perimenopause because:

- Perimenopause is a time in which hormones fluctuate significantly, which can feel destabilizing.

- Hormonal imbalances can increase anxiety, depression and rage.

- Some women experience uncomfortable symptoms during perimenopause, including lack of sleep, which can affect their mood.

You may experience symptoms, including:

- Feelings of sadness.

- Irritability (one study found 70 percent of women cite irritability as the most common symptom they experience in perimenopause[66]).

- Lack of motivation.

---

66 Born, Leslie et al. "A new, female-specific irritability rating scale." *Journal of psychiatry & neuroscience: JPN* vol. 33,4 (2008): 344–354.

- Anxiety.

- Aggressiveness.

- Difficulty concentrating.

- Mood changes.

- Fatigue.

- Tension.

In fact, in a recent study of 40,000 women in menopause, 60 percent experienced anxiety and depression[67].

Hot Tip: Keep in mind that if you have experienced bad PMS throughout your life, you are more likely to experience rage during perimenopause. That's because estrogen affects the production of serotonin, which is a mood regulator and happiness booster, and our bodies produce less estrogen in perimenopause.

TIPS FOR MANAGING SYMPTOMS

I have said this so many times in this guide so far so at this point it will seem repetitive, but your first step should be: *test your hormones.* Why?

- Many women, including myself, become depressed in perimenopause due to an undiagnosed thyroid condition.

---

67   Megan McGibney, "Perimenopause can trigger high anxiety. Nobody told these women that it's normal." *The Lily*, November 2021.

- Lots and lots of women describe anxiety as the first symptom of perimenopause. That's because their "feel calm" progesterone has bottomed out.

- Many women become depressed because they're exhausted from lack of sleep due to hot flashes caused by low estrogen levels.

- Lots and lots of women experience periods of rage during perimenopause because of imbalances between estrogen and serotonin.

In other words, balancing your hormones should be the first step to addressing any emotional and mental health symptoms because it very well could be your hormones that are causing mental and emotional issues.

A number of other remedies and lifestyle approaches can also help with mental and emotional challenges, including:

- **Exercise.** Exercising can release serotonin and endorphins into our bodies, both of which may help with anxiety and depression. This does not need to be a "killer workout"! Walking has helped me enormously manage my mental health. There's something about walking that I find very soothing and adding upbeat music to my walks never fails to shift my perspective when I need it. See Chapter 11 for in-depth details on moving our bodies in perimenopause.

- **Sleep.** Make sure you are getting good sleep. My advice is to aim for seven to nine hours of uninterrupted sleep every night. Try to go bed at the same time every night in a quiet, dark, cool room and avoid using electronics in bed. See Chapter 11 for more sleeping beauty tips.

- **Medication Can Make a Difference. Talk with Your Care Team.** Many of us were born with brain chemistries that predispose us to depression, anxiety and other mental and emotional conditions. I believe strongly that some brain chemistries require medication and that it is impossible to achieve a healthy mental state without medication. With that said, as I was writing this guide, I was very disturbed by the number of women who told me their clinicians prescribed antidepression and antianxiety medication in perimenopause without testing their hormones. This tells me some of us may be on medications for issues that could easily be taken care of by balancing our hormones or getting enough sleep. If you are experiencing anxiety or depression for the first time in perimenopause, make sure your care team tests your hormones and shares hormone balancing options with you before prescribing other medications.

- **B Vitamins: Another Powerful Tool.** As I mentioned earlier in this guide, serotonin levels fluctuate in perimenopause and may lead to mood swings, depression and rage. Vitamins B6 and B12 play an important role in the creation of serotonin, so aim to include vitamin B–rich food in your diet (see Chapter 10 for more information on eating for hormone balance in perimenopause). Supplements can also help provide the Vitamin B needed in perimenopause. I use the **Nature's Bounty** brand sublingual Vitamin B12.

- **Reduce stress and anxiety.** Life seems to move at a million miles an hour these days. We all have long to-do lists and not enough time to get them done. For many of us, a fast-paced life leads to stress and anxiety. Others of us are parenting, caring for elder adults and working. I know many of us also deal with generalized anxiety disorder, which is exacerbated in perimenopause due to hormone shifts. It's a lot. I'm including next the top two things that have helped me reduce stress and anxiety in perimenopause.

1. **Mindfulness.** Years ago, I happened upon a book called *Wherever You Go, There You Are* by Jon Kabat-Zin. The book is focused on mindfulness, and it may seem like an exaggeration, but that book changed my life. Mindfulness is the intentional act of paying attention to the present moment without judgment. During a mindfulness practice, you are encouraged to notice and accept your thoughts and feelings without trying to change them. Mindfulness helped me slow down as I go about my fast-paced life. In a recent study of perimenopausal women, those who had higher mindfulness scores reported fewer menopausal symptoms.[68] Since I read Jon Kabat-Zin's book, he has created a mindfulness-based stress reduction program that you can learn about at the Mindfulness Studies (MBSR) website: www. mindfulnessstudies.com/personal. Bonus: women who completed an eight-week MBSR course reported a 39 percent reduction in hot flash symptoms.[69]

---

68   Mayo Clinic. "Mindfulness may ease menopausal symptoms." ScienceDaily, 17 January 2019. www.sciencedaily.com/releases/2019/01/190117090449.htm.

69   Carmody, James Francis et al. "Mindfulness training for coping with hot flashes: Results of a randomized trial." *Menopause* (New York) vol. 18,6 (2011): 611–620. doi:10.1097/gme.0b013e318204a05c

2. **Meditation.** Jon Kabat-Zin's book also introduced me to the world of meditation, which has been shown to help reduce stress and anxiety. In fact, according to the Cleveland Clinic, while research on the benefits of meditation is ongoing, existing research indicates a regular meditation practice can also help "improve sleep, improve pain management ... improve self-esteem, improve concentration" and even "decrease menopausal symptoms, and reduce the severity of symptoms of irritable bowel syndrome." Over the years I've done Zen and transcendental meditation, both of which have helped me enormously in regulating my emotions and managing stress. If you are interested in learning more about Zen Buddhism and meditation, I recommend checking out the Tricycle Foundation at https://tricycle. org/about. If you are interested in learning more about transcendental meditation, I recommend checking out the David Lynch Foundation at www.davidlynchfoundation.org/about-tm.html. There are also tons of meditation apps available including **Calm** and **Headspace**, both of which I highly recommend.

My wish for everyone reading this guide is that you will not experience mental and emotional challenges in perimenopause. However, it's important to know mental and emotional challenges do occur for many women in perimenopause and it's important to:

- Know what those challenges might be.

- Know what options exist to help you manage your mental and emotional health in perimenopause.

Chapter 14.

FLIP THE SCRIPT ON PERIMENOPAUSE

> **"I MAY BE IN THE MINORITY, BUT I'VE FOUND**
> perimenopause somewhat liberating. I think it started for me in my
> mid-forties. I've built up years of wisdom at work, so I feel more
> confident in my career than ever before. I also feel more centered
> and secure in myself, maybe because I finally have time to devote
> to myself. I use that time to exercise and I've started playing the
> piano again. It's amazing what a little time to yourself can do! It
> seems like the hardest years of parenting are behind me, which
> is a relief, and my husband and I are able to focus more on our
> relationship. I've dealt with some frustrating physical symptoms
> but overall, it's been a good time for me and I'm really looking
> forward to being done with a monthly period." — *Farinaz*

I want to share a fundamental belief I have. I believe it so strongly that it spurred me to write this guide in the first place. You can thrive in perimenopause. There is so much unknown about perimenopause that it can seem scary. Not to mention that perimenopause has the word *menopause* in it and many of us have been hearing whispers of the horrors of menopause our entire lives. I'm here to tell you peri-menopause doesn't have to be a nightmare. It's time to flip the script.

PERIMENOPAUSE MEANS MIDLIFE

Historically, perimenopause and menopause have been associated with old age because when our great-great grandmothers were in per-imenopause, women's life expectancy was fifty, maybe sixty years old. That meant perimenopause did in some ways signal old age because tour great-great grandmothers likely only had twenty or so years to live when it arrived. Today, however, women's life expectancy is approxi-mately eighty-one years old (variations exist by race, state etc.). Lots of us will begin perimenopause in our mid-forties, which means we have about another forty years to live. To me, perimenopause signals mid-life, meaning I hopefully have another forty years to go on adventures, spend time with family, and make an impact in the world. Bring it on!

I mention this because as you likely know, many cultures around the world worship youth whereas older people are devalued and even become invisible—metaphorically and literally if they are in nursing homes cut off from the world. Additionally, it often feels as though as women we are most valued in our reproductive years and are viewed as least valuable to society as we age. I don't know about you, but this phenomenon is both frustrating and hurtful! None of us want to be written off that way, and given how many years are ahead for many of us, I feel it's important to begin shifting thinking about perimenopause.

GET RID OF OUTDATED THINKING

The way we think about perimenopause today is influenced by our past, when most medical research was done on men, ignoring the physiological and hormonal issues unique to women. Without medical data to explain physical or emotional symptoms, communities came up with their own explanations, often negative ones. For example, women in perimenopause and menopause were labeled "hysterical" or "mad"—otherwise known as insane. In other words, instead of perimenopause and menopause being viewed as natural stages of life, historically, they have been seen and treated as something negative to be eradicated or downright ignored. We don't have to accept this thinking. We can change how we feel and talk about perimenopause, and we can change the stigma associated with perimenopause for ourselves and for our nieces, daughters and granddaughters who will come after us.

LISTEN FOR DIFFERENT EXPERIENCES

In addition to the historical baggage associated with perimenopause, very few of us have heard stories or anecdotes from women about their positive or even neutral perimenopause and menopause experiences. This means for many of us there's no new shared narrative to replace the old one. With that said, I interviewed many women, and these are some of the things they shared with me:

- "I'm enjoying perimenopause. My periods are lighter than they've ever been, and I no longer get cramps every month."

- "I've been very fortunate not to have any symptoms at all in perimenopause. I don't have any issues or concerns and I can't wait for menopause and the end of a monthly period."

- "I'm in menopause now and if I could tell my younger self anything I would tell her to hang on, life keeps getting better and better."

These experiences are not unusual. In fact, a Gennev survey of women in perimenopause and postmenopause found the majority of women felt better about life now than they did ten years prior.[70] So, there you go! For many women, not only is perimenopause *not* a nightmare, it's the beginning of a new and better stage of our lives.

LOOK FOR THE POSITIVES

Despite the fact that early perimenopause was tough for me, one thing I appreciate about this stage of life is that my self-confidence has increased. Maybe it is because as I get older I have fewer @$%s to give. Maybe it's because I have learned mistakes happen and that's where the lessons are. I'm not certain why my self-confidence has increased, but friends have shared similar sentiments with me. They tell me they have learned a lot about the importance of healthy boundaries in the first forty years of their lives and now in perimenopause they are no longer willing to compromise on those boundaries. These friends are more likely to push back at work when given assignments with unrealistic deadlines, for example. They are unwilling to stay silent with family members about issues that matter to them or needs they have.

Perimenopause may be the nudge we need to leave an unfulfilling job or let go of a friendship that no longer feels right. We may relish that empty-nesting is ahead of us. Some of us may begin planning for a time when we can downshift our careers a bit and look forward to having more time to spend with family and friends or have more hours in the day to devote to hobbies. Others of us may be looking forward to going back to school and finishing our degrees. One woman shared with me that perimenopause is the first time in her life she has the time and energy to understand who she is and what she wants. The bottom

---

70   https://gennev.com/education/menopause-statistics-zeitgeist

line is that today's perimenopause can look and feel very differently than what our great-great grandmothers experienced. So, rather than viewing perimenopause as a dreaded stage of life with lots of challenges, let's look for the positives. There are plenty of positives, but we may need practice finding them. Read on for more!

MAKE YOUR BRAIN WORK FOR YOU

Okay, now that we know the perimenopause script that was given to us is a load of crap, let's look at the role our brain plays in perimenopause. Why? Because we're in control of two things: our minds and the way we talk to ourselves. Here's the thing, even though the script is outdated (big time!), many of us will experience negative physical and emotional symptoms during perimenopause. I've shared strategies in other parts of this guide for managing these symptoms, but mindset plays a big part as well. In fact, our thoughts have tremendous power. In a number of studies, researchers found women who viewed menopause in more negative terms reported more frequent and severe physical symptoms; whereas women who viewed menopause in a more positive light reported fewer and less severe symptoms.[71] Granted these studies are about menopause, but I imagine the same is true for perimenopause. When it comes to perimenopause, of all of the factors that influence our experience, we have the most control over our personal mindset. So, let's do something about it!

OUR MINDS

It's not something I advertise or talk a lot about with friends, but I'm a huge neuroscience geek. I've spent hours upon hours reading

---

71 Yanikkerem E, Koltan SO, Tamay AG, Dikayak Ş. Relationship between women's attitude towards menopause and quality of life. Climacteric. 2012 Dec;15(6):552–562. doi: 10.3109/13697137.2011.637651. Epub 2012 Feb 15. PMID: 22335298

neuroscience books and medical literature. Human behavior fascinates me, and neuroscience is the science that focuses on the brain and its impact on behavioral and cognitive functions, or how people think. One of the things I've learned from neuroscience is that while our senses are automatic (we smell, taste, and hear not with thought, but reflexively), our perceptions are not. This is an amazing thing because that means we can influence and change our perceptions. This is known as neuroplasticity and it's downright cool. Neuroplasticity refers to the brain's ability to modify itself. The process involves different neurochemicals and it's all pretty complicated, so I won't go into great detail here. What I do want to share is two concepts that I have not only read about but I have observed in myself.

1. **What We Focus on Expands and We Tend to Focus on the Negative.** As humans we are wired to notice threats and bad feelings. It's what kept us from being eaten by tigers in the savannah thousands of years ago. Our brains are very good at paying attention to negative things, analyzing those things and hanging onto everything associated with them until we have learned something useful to our survival. Not only that, but what we notice becomes what we think and what we think becomes our experience. Here's an example:

   - **Focus.** "I'm noticing I'm more tired in perimenopause."

   - **Brain.** "Perimenopause is a negative thing that results in being more tired."

   - **Body.** "I'm tired."

2. **We Are Not Wired to Notice and Hold on to Positive Things.** For example, rather than remembering numerous compliments we receive from colleagues, we are more likely to recall

the one negative piece of feedback shared with us. This means we have to be intentional about focusing on the positive as a way to counteract the negative. This takes work because we're going against our brain's natural instincts. However, based on personal experience, I know intentionally focusing on the positive works and it makes a difference. When I was first in perimenopause I focused only on symptoms that were causing me frustration and I was miserable. I woke up miserable and I went to bed miserable. At one point I decided I need to change my mindset or it was going to be a long and miserable ten years. I started to list out the positives associated with perimenopause:

- "I get to supplement with progesterone. No more heavy periods or monthly cramps. Yay!"

- "I'm treating myself to some seriously decadent body cream: go me!"

- "I slept like a baby last night thanks to that Valerian I took. Nice!"

I focused on these positives and over time as I found my own perimenopause dream team, the list of positives grew longer and longer. Here's the thing: all of our thoughts release some type of chemical. Positive thoughts produce serotonin, a feel-good chemical. Dopamine may also be released if we feel pleasure. Negative thoughts produce the stress hormones cortisol and adrenalin. If you've learned anything in this book so far, it is that *hormones are everything*. Balancing them is a challenge and the last thing we want is more of the stress hormones. It's important to control our mindset.

IT'S NOT ABOUT TOXIC POSITIVITY

I don't want this section to be misunderstood as me pedaling toxic positivity. That's not my intent at all. In fact, I believe strongly that it's important for all of us to:

- Feel our feelings. Don't ignore or deny them. Feelings are important.

- Come to terms with our feelings. Acknowledge them and share them with others if it's helpful or gives us relief.

Adopting a positive mindset is in no way, shape or form denying our experience or our feelings. However, it is a way to manage our brain when we're dealing with a challenging time or experience (and not challenging times too). It breaks my heart to think of anyone feeling miserable for ten years of perimenopause, so try and take charge your brain because you really have nothing to lose.

OUR INTERNAL VOICE

Now that I've addressed the power of our minds to influence our experiences, let me talk about our internal voice because our internal voice both informs and reflects our mind. I suffer from mind chatter like you read about despite years of meditating and chanting. If I'm not meditating or talking out loud, my brain is talking, talking, talking. I know I'm not alone. It's the human condition to have a nonstop voice chatting in our heads so I don't try to stop my chatter because it's pointless. Instead, what I've learned to do through meditation is to observe that chatter. I observe it because the words I use and the things I say to myself are directly related to how I'm feeling about myself, others and my experiences. Those feelings then influence my future experiences. So, once I know those feelings, I can gently reframe the most negative of them. As I've shared in this guide, I beat myself up a lot when I first entered perimenopause.

- **Me:** "Wow, I'm really weak. I can't lift weights like I used to."

- **Me:** "Ugh, I never get anything done because I'm always tired."

It took me a little while, but I slowly started reframing those thoughts.

- **Me:** "I may not be lifting what I used to, but I showed up today. I'm getting stronger every day."

- **Me:** "Sleep is important to me and my health. I'm making it a priority even if other things or other people's needs have to wait."

The trick with mind chatter is to not beat yourself up when you can't reframe negative thoughts. Here's a classic run-through of what I mean.

- **Me:** "I forgot my thyroid medication today like an idiot. Now I'm going to be exhausted all day."

- **Also Me:** "Stop calling yourself an idiot. You're always so negative."

- **Also Me:** "Omg, I can't believe anyone is letting me write a book on anything. I can't even stop my own negative self-talk!"

Holy brain spiral! I'm sharing this because it's a true story and I hope it made you laugh! I want to emphasize that it can take some time to hone the reframe process and, like me, you may have some bumps along the way. That's totally normal! Keep trying. If you continue to struggle to reframe your negative self-talk, I highly recommend looking into cognitive behavioral therapy (CBT), which is a specific way of reframing negative thought patterns. Bonus: CBT is recommended by the North American Society for Menopause as an effective treatment for hot flashes and night sweats. In one study, women who participated in eight hours of CBT reported a 50 percent reduction in hot flashes and night sweats—which is about as effective as HRT.[72]

Let's recap: it's not surprising that some of us may worry about or be fearful of perimenopause given the negative things we have heard and the stigmas associated with it. Some of us have heard nothing about perimenopause and that silence alone can be worrisome. I hope this chapter has helped shift your mindset on perimenopause to see we can actually thrive in perimenopause. In fact, many women do! If I have learned anything in my time on this planet, it is that women can accomplish anything. I truly believe that by being intentional about taking charge of our thoughts and ensuring our internal voice is not sabotaging us, we can all flip the outdated perimenopause script.

---

72   Hunter M, Rendall M. Bio-psycho-socio-cultural perspectives on menopause. *Best Pract Res Clin Obstet Gynaecol* 2007;21:261–274.

Chapter 15:

NAVIGATING SEX & INTIMACY: IT'S COMPLICATED

> **"A COUPLE OF YEARS AGO, I STARTED TO** notice a new 'odor' to my vagina. I've always been attuned to my body and I have no hang-ups regarding body smells, but this smell felt both 'new' and 'off' and frankly, it made me worried about being intimate with my partner. Let's just say, my sex life hasn't been great lately. — *Valeria*

A couple of years ago, one of my girlfriends shared that she started "drying up down there." At one point, she semi-joked she felt like she was growing sandpaper in her vagina. Well, you can imagine how unappealing sex sounded to her while her vagina felt like sandpaper! Unfortunately for me, she was not alone. In the early days of perimenopause, I found intercourse very uncomfortable due to increasing vaginal dryness, which is one of the most common symptoms of perimenopause.

In advance of writing this guide, I spoke with, interviewed, and surveyed lots of women. Many, many, many (many!) of them told me their sex drives had completely tanked. They simply had zero interest in sex. Some of these women didn't miss sex, and lack of sex with their partners had no effect on their relationship with their partners. They were, however, the minority. The vast majority told me they miss having an active sex life, they're frustrated that even when they do have sex it's less satisfying, and in some cases uncomfortable, and they are concerned their decreasing sex drives are affecting their relationships negatively.

The other themes I heard over and over again in my interviews were:

- "If perimenopause happened to men, the world would have figured out solutions a long time ago."

- "It's like no one seems to know or care about women's sex drives. They only care about men and their ability to have an erection."

As I listened to these women, it was clear to me that sex in perimenopause is a weighted subject with lots of emotion attached to it. Many of us feel that as women we have been let down, our needs not prioritized and our concerns discounted. I'd like to say this very clearly (and if I were with you in person I might lean in for emphasis and even increase the sound of my voice a little for effect): *You have every right to a satisfying sexual relationship with your partner(s) before perimenopause, during perimenopause, in menopause, and after menopause.*

It's not your fault many cultures have baggage when it comes to women's sexuality. I'm not going to expand on that baggage because that would be a book in and of itself. But I will say I'm with you. I'm disappointed by how little information is available to women to help us manage perimenopause generally, and especially to manage any changes in our sex lives in particular. It's one of the reasons I decided to write this guide. I've learned and already shared some things from my perimenopause journey that I hope will help you. This guide may not have all the answers about sex during this stage of life, though, so just as I have in other parts of this book, I encourage you to find a health-care team that specializes in hormone balancing and will work with you to uncover solutions that work for you, your needs and your body.

Let's break down a couple of things about sex and perimenopause. First, perimenopause represents two things many cultures don't value: aging and decreasing fertility. In cultures that worship youth and fertility, perimenopause is a set-up for women to feel badly about ourselves. That's an issue, isn't it? We feel like we're being told we're less desirable, valued etc.

Let's break things down a little farther. There's a sense in our culture that as we get older we no longer have interest in sex. Where does that come from? Well, it could be true! Perhaps our desire does decrease due to a decrease in the hormones that govern our sexual desire.

- But what if it isn't true? What if our desire remains the same but our bodies don't work the way they used to?

- Or what if it's true and it leaves us sad and frustrated? What if we mourn the loss of our sex drive or are frustrated by changes in our bodies?

- What if we anticipate living another forty years and want to preserve our sex lives—a key dimension of our happiness?

This leads to the million-dollar question: In 2021, in a world with cutting-edge medicine at our finger tips, with potentially forty more years ahead of many of us, does it have to be this way?

I know from personal experience it doesn't have to be, and I also know from speaking with many other women that my experience is not unique. As I shared in Chapter 7, taking bio-identical hormones was an absolute game changer for me when it came to perimenopause. What I didn't share in that chapter was that in addition to helping me with perimenopause symptoms, bio-identical hormones also over-hauled my sex life. Why? Because my hormones were balanced. What this meant was I went from feeling dry everywhere (yes, I'm referring to my vagina, but also my forehead all the way down to the bottom of my feet) to having moisture return to my body. Most importantly, my sex drive returned and sex was enjoyable once again. So how do hormones affect your sex life during perimenopause? Let's break them down one by one:

MAJOR SEX HORMONES

Estrogen

Estrogen is one of the hormone "stars" of the show when it comes to sexual desire and experience. Typically, our sex drive is highest at points in our menstrual cycle when our estrogen levels are highest. That's because estrogen can be energizing. You may even find that your skin glows and your hair is shinier when your estrogen levels peak in your cycle.

Estrogen is made up of three components: estradiol, estriol and estrone. During our reproductive years, the majority of our estrogen is made up of estradiol. As we age, our estradiol decreases and if it gets too low, our vagina gets dry, which of course can make sex painful and intimacy a challenge. Additionally, lower levels of estrogen can result in decreased blood supply to the vagina, which may cause the nerve sensors in the clitoris and labia minora (your inner vagina) to become less responsive. You may find it harder to orgasm, and when you do, it could be barely perceptible. Not cool!

Low estrogen, aka estradiol, is also frequently the culprit for both hot flashes and insomnia. I know I speak for many women when I say nothing kills interest in sex more than being exhausted, which is what many of us are dealing with between insomnia and hot flashes that awaken us in the middle of the night.

Finally, low estrogen can result in loss of bladder control. This may happen when we sneeze or it can happen when we jump on a trampoline. It can also happen just by walking slowly into a room. Some women experience loss of bladder control after pregnancy, but others only experience this symptom as estrogen decreases in peri-menopause. I know I'm not alone when I say feeling like I can't fully control my bladder would definitely have an impact on my sexual desire. Bottom line: low estrogen can do a number on sex and intimacy in perimenopause.

Progesterone

At first glance, it might seem like progesterone does not play a signif-icant role in sex drive or sexual pleasure. As I've described in other sections of this guide, progesterone is the "feel good" hormone. It helps us to feel balanced and can stave off stress. On the flip side, progester-one can make us feel bloated and sluggish. Premenstrual syndrome is a result of an increase in progesterone levels. You may also notice that your sex drive decreases toward the end of your cycle. That's because estrogen levels decrease and progesterone increases toward the end of your cycle.

As I shared in Chapter 4, it's imperative that progesterone and estrogen work together to maintain hormone balance. Progesterone can become problematic when its levels are higher than our estrogen levels, which is the main hormone when it comes to sex drive and sexual pleasure. When that's the case, our sex drive decreases. At the same time, too little progesterone can impact sleep, mood and our ability to think (i.e., we get brain fog), all of which can influence both our interest in and our experience with sex. At this point in this guide, it should not surprise you to hear that it's a delicate dance keeping hormone levels in balance, particularly estrogen and progesterone, and being in balance is what we're aiming for if having a satisfying sex life is a priority.

Testosterone

Testosterone is the sex hormone most associated with men, but it has a significant role in women's sexual health too. Testosterone is *the* hormone of desire, meaning it's the hormone that makes us want to have sex. Testosterone is also key to sexual responsiveness and sensitivity. Your ability to orgasm or lack thereof is directly tied to testosterone levels. Additionally, balanced testosterone levels contribute to the thickness of your vaginal tissues. Thick vaginal tissues mean more pleasurable intercourse whereas thinner vaginal walls mean the vagina is drier, and less elastic or flexible. Testosterone also increases energy, stabilizes mood and can improve self-confidence and self-esteem, all of which can make a huge difference in our interest in and experience of sex and intimacy. Finally, testosterone can offset some of the symptoms of decreasing estrogen levels like hot flashes and vaginal dryness. In other words: testosterone is very important to sex and intimacy!

While estrogen and progesterone levels decrease quickly during perimenopause and menopause, specifically, testosterone levels decrease gradually as we age. Some women, however, may experience a significant decrease in testosterone levels if they have their ovaries removed due to ovarian cysts or if they undergo a hysterectomy. Testosterone levels can also be affected by birth control pills. That's because in women, testosterone is created partially in the ovaries. Birth control pills turn our ovaries "off," which lowers testosterone production and levels. If you noticed your sex drive diminish while on birth control pills, they could be the culprit.

Some of us will not notice any symptoms as our testosterone levels fall as we age. Others of us may be surprised and concerned by plummeting sexual interest due to lower testosterone levels. The challenge with testosterone is similar to the challenge of estrogen and progesterone levels, which is that the levels are unique to each of us and they must all be in balance for us to feel our best emotionally, mentally and physically.

People are very surprised when they learn I do testosterone replacement therapy. I had never heard of such a thing and neither had 99 percent of my friends and family. I had seen "low-T" commercials, but I only associated the condition with senior men, not women in their mid-forties. The irony for me is that I'm not a muscular person at all, which is what many of us associate with testosterone. In fact, my sisters and I have joked for years that we don't have the muscle-making gene. However, the decline in testosterone levels was obvious to me pretty quickly because my previously healthy and enjoyable interest in and experience of sex disappeared. Gone, poof! As best as I can surmise, my already low testosterone levels decreased as I entered midlife and also as I struggled with estrogen dominance.

One More (Minor) Sex Hormone (but Still Important)

Oxytocin

Oxytocin is sometimes referred to as the love hormone. After a baby is born, for example, both women and men release large amounts of oxytocin, which helps them bond with the newborn baby. Oxytocin is also released when women breastfeed, helping them relax and fall in love with their child. Oxytocin is a power player in that it's not just important post childbirth. Oxytocin relieves anxiety, it helps us feel happy and loving and it also helps women feel orgasms.

Oxytocin may also play a role in progesterone regulation. The signals received by the ovaries to produce progesterone in the second half of the menstrual cycle may be delivered by oxytocin. Estrogen stimulates the production of oxytocin and as estrogen levels decrease, women's levels of oxytocin decrease as well, which can leave us feeling anxious, less happy and less likely to feel our orgasms. Not okay!

HORMONE REPLACEMENT THERAPY

If you suspect hormones may be playing a role in your decreased sex drive or affecting the degree to which you experience sex as plea-surable, I recommend working with a care team that specializes in hormone balancing. They will test your hormones and they can recommend hormone replacement therapies to address any issues you may be experiencing. I wrote about hormone balancing options in great detail in Chapter 7, so while I won't repeat myself here, I want to say a couple of things about how it applies to sex and intimacy, specifically:

1. I separated out sex and intimacy into its own chapter because some of us may pay more attention to other symptoms but blow off any symptoms related to our sex drives and sexual experiences as "just perimenopause." I think declining sex

drive or less pleasurable sexual experiences as we age are very worthy of our attention and I hope this guide plays a part in normalizing that idea.

2. For some women, a change in their sexual desire or sexual pleasure is the only symptom of perimenopause they experience. I want to make sure all of you who fall into this camp know it's okay to be disappointed in those symptoms and want to do something about them even if you're sailing through the rest of the perimenopause experience.

3. Hormone replacement therapy can require patience and some trial and error to "dial in" the right treatment and to minimize any side effects associated with treatment. That is true when it comes to hot flashes and it's even more true when it comes to sexual desire. For example, it can take up to six months for some women to notice positive changes with their sexual desire due to hormone replacement. Other women find that while their desire increases, they cannot tolerate the side effects they experience, like acne. My advice is to start slowly, test after six weeks to understand how your body is responding to the replacement therapy and always test your hormone levels prior to re-dosing.

4. I'll be honest, I've been frustrated for a long time at the ways many cultures appear to prioritize male sexual needs and satisfaction over female sexual needs and satisfaction. Viagra: need I say more? My hope is that more women will share with their clinicians the concerns they have about the ways in which their desires and experiences have changed during perimenopause. That sharing could lead to more clinical research on perimenopause and a greater range of treatments

and therapies available to all of us. Which brings us to the next section.

NON-HORMONE-REPLACEMENT OPTIONS

My hope is that this guide will help women see that hormone replacement can be a safe, viable option in perimenopause. With that said, I recognize and fully respect that some women will not feel comfortable with HRT, so I include in what follows some information on alternatives I have gathered on this topic. Keep in mind that while I am sharing with you the research I did, you must do your own due diligence as I am not a medical professional or an herbalist. Additionally, if you choose to take any of these remedies, please be transparent with your health-care providers in order to avoid any dangerous medication combinations or issues.

According to my research, there are only two herbal remedies to address changes in sexual desire and experience that have double-blind research studies demonstrating their efficacy. ArginMax and Zestra are described next.

ArginMax

ArginMax is a blend of L-arginine, ginseng, ginkgo and damiana, plus multivitamins and minerals. The herbal components of ArginMax are thought to improve sexual satisfaction by increasing blood flow and by promoting muscle relaxation. Small studies have shown that ArginMax can improve sexual function in both women and men. For example, one double-blind, placebo-controlled study published in 2006, showed

ArginMax to significantly improve levels of sexual desire and sex life satisfaction in 68% of women in four weeks.[73]

IMPORTANT NOTE: Patients with hormone-sensitive cancers should be careful as ginseng has estrogenic effects. The L-Arginine can make symptoms worse in people with asthma. It can also affect blood sugar, therefore people with diabetes should be careful when using this product. Ginseng and ginkgo can cause interactions with other prescription drugs. So again, check with your health-care provider.

Zestra

Zestra contains borage seed oil, evening primrose oil, angelica rose extract, Coleaus forskohlii extract, ascorbyl palmitate and dl-alpha tocopherol and is used to address sexual function issues including painful intercourse, loss of desire and difficulty in achieving arousal or orgasm. A small study suggests Zestra can improve sexual function in both healthy women and in those suffering from female sexual arousal disorder.[74]

While extensive research has not been done on Maca or medicinal mushrooms, I have used them both for temporary relief of sexual

---

73 Ito TY, Polan ML, Whipple B, Trant AS. The enhancement of female sexual function with ArginMax, a nutritional supplement, among women differing in menopausal status. J Sex Marital Ther. 2006 Oct–Dec;32(5):369–78. doi: 10.1080/00926230600834901. PMID: 16959660

74 Ferguson DM, Steidle CP, Singh GS, Alexander JS, Weihmiller MK, Crosby MG. Randomized, placebo-controlled, double blind, crossover design trial of the efficacy and safety of Zestra for Women in women with and without female sexual arousal disorder. J Sex Marital Ther. 2003;29 Suppl 1:33–44. doi: 10.1080/713847125. PMID: 1273

dysfunction with good success. I share some information below on them in case they're interesting options for you.

Maca

Maca is a plant native to the Andes mountain range that is known as an adaptogen. Adaptogens are natural substances that help the body adapt to stress and help the body normalize and balance its processes. For the best-quality product, look for organic maca grown in Peru. It is believed that maca can enhance sex drive, increase energy levels and sexual fertility and increase blood flow to the vagina. While it is not completely understood how maca works, research demonstrates it may offset the sexual side effects women experience when they take antidepressants. Those side effects include low libido, vaginal dryness and difficulty reaching orgasm.[75] Because it is not clear how maca affects hormones, it is not advised to take maca if you have one of the following conditions:

- Breast, uterine, or ovarian cancer.

- Endometriosis.

- Uterine fibroids.

- Thyroid disease.

Medical Mushrooms

Known in the West as Cordyceps sinensis, "medical mush-rooms" have been used for thousands of years by Tibetans, Nepalese, Chinese and many other cultures as potent natural aphrodisi-acs. Cordyceps sinensis is an adaptogen herb believed to increase

---

75   Evidence-Based Complementary and Alternative Medicine Volume 2015, Article ID 949036, 9 pages http://dx.doi.org/10.1155/2015/949036

testosterone properties, thereby increasing sexual desire and drive. Cordyceps sinensis is also believed to increase energy levels and aid our bodies in dealing with stress.

IMPORTANT NOTE (and I know I'm repeating myself): Herbal supplements aren't monitored by the FDA the same way medications are. You can't always be certain of what you're getting and whether it's safe. Herbal supplement contents may not be consistent and may include other ingredients. Remember, natural doesn't always mean safe. When selecting a brand of supplements, look for products that have been third-party tested and contain safe levels of vitamins and minerals.

TALKING WITH YOUR CARE TEAM

It's highly ironic that I'm writing a guide with an entire chapter on sex and intimacy because as I mentioned earlier in this guide, I didn't grow up with a high level of comfort with these topics. I didn't even have the appropriate biological terminology available to me until I went to college, and my family certainly didn't speak about these topics openly. I have a feeling some of you can relate! I've watched over the past forty years as there appears to be more and more openness about the topic of sexuality and yet I think it can still feel like a "charged" or embarrassing topic for many of us. This is a challenge because embarrassment prevents many women from seeking help. I hope reading this guide will give you the motivation and knowledge to speak up.

To help, I include in what follows some specific language you can use when speaking to your care team about sex and intimacy during perimenopause. Keep in mind, clinicians have spent years studying and treating human bodies. Many of them have seen it all, so don't be shy. With that said, if anyone on your care team shows even the *slightest* level of discomfort about talking about these topics, makes you feel ashamed in any way or is dismissive about your questions or concerns, *find a different care team.*

Things to Share

- *I'm concerned my sex drive is diminishing. I don't desire sex as often as I used to. Why would that be? What are my options?*

- *I've noticed my vagina is dry, which is uncomfortable and makes intercourse painful/not enjoyable. What are my options?*

- *My partner and I are still having sex but I can't really feel anything. I'm not having orgasms the way I used to. How can I change that?*

- *I feel anxious all of the time, very tense and less joyful, which means I have no interest in being intimate with my partner. Why is that? What can I do about it?*

MAYBE IT'S NOT THE HORMONES

While it can be tempting to believe perimenopause is the culprit for any and all physical or emotional changes you may be experiencing, that is not always the case, especially when it comes to sexual desire and satisfaction. As you prepare for perimenopause, it's important to track your hormone levels regularly as well as pay attention to these other factors:

Stress

Leslie, one of the women I spoke with as I was writing this guide, shared with me the following: "My sex life dried up while I wasn't paying attention." She explained that as a busy entrepreneur she was constantly under stress. She was running her business managing many aspects of her parents' transition to an assisted living facility. Leslie's personal needs, like exercise and eating healthfully, were no longer a priority and a fulfilling sex life had completely fallen off the list of priorities.

Leslie's story is not unique. Many of us are stressed to a breaking point these days and our sex lives pay the price. It's not just that sex falls off of our to-do lists, but for many of us, desire disappears when we're stressed and stress impacts the degree to which we feel pleasure when we do have sex. My sense is that we all assume being stressed is inevitable. Please make it a habit to monitor your stress levels and aim to establish a habit of one or two regular stress-relieving activities. Check out Chapters 11 and 13 for some of the ways I have reduced my stress with success.

Anxiety and Depression

General anxiety and depression levels are off the charts in the United States (nearly 50 percent of adults say they have experienced anxiety or depression in the past year[76]). The COVID-19 pandemic has only increased those levels. Anxiety of any kind can result in decreased interest in sex because when we're anxious, we have higher cortisol (our body's main stress hormone) levels, which can suppress the sex hormones that play a role in desire. Some of us may feel anxious about physical changes we're seeing or feeling in our bodies during

---

76   www.cdc.gov/mmwr/volumes/70/wr/mm7013e2.htm

perimenopause and those anxious feelings may dampen our desire or feelings of desirability. Others of us may continue to desire sex, but we're so anxious that we can't relax enough to enjoy intimacy or to orgasm. As my friend Lena shared with me: "I'm calculating college costs in my head before bed every night, which makes it really hard to actually enjoy sex." Depression can also impact our sex lives. Not only can depression negatively impact our sex drive but many of the medications that treat depression reduce sex drive. If you are experiencing anxiety or depression, work with your care team to address your symptoms and if you are concerned about any treatments affecting your sex drive or intimacy with your partner, share those concerns.

Your Relationship

Midlife is a time when many of us examine our intimate relationships, and sometimes they come up short. Not surprisingly, if you are not getting what you need from your partner or your relationship is rife with conflict, it's highly likely your libido and experience of sex itself will be affected. Bottom line: no amount of hormone replacement or other remedies can or should replace a loving, connected relationship with your partner.

Alcohol and Drugs

I wrote quite a bit about alcohol use in Chapter 10, but I did not address its effect on sex and intimacy. The reality is that despite what movies, television and social media tell us, alcohol and drugs are more likely to negatively impact our sex drive and experience of sex than to enhance them in any way. If you find your evening wine habit has gotten out of control at the same time your sex drive has tanked, it could be the wine.

A FINAL THOUGHT

I'll end this chapter the way I began it. We all deserve to have enjoyable and fulfilling sex lives, if we desire that—even (and perhaps especially) in perimenopause and menopause. My goal is that this section of the guide affirms that for you. My wish is that the suggestions here help you achieve whatever hopes you have for sex and intimacy in midlife.

Chapter 16:

WE'RE ALL ADULTS HERE: TALKING ABOUT PERIMENOPAUSE

> **"THE BEST THING I EVER DID WAS SIT MY** partner down and tell her what I was going through. She's ten years younger than me and I went through perimenopause early, so even though we're both women, she was completely clueless. She could tell I was struggling but she had never even heard of perimenopause let alone knew what it was. I felt such relief finally just saying the word 'perimenopause.' Up until then I worried it would make me sound old, but the reality is I need her support and it's nothing to be ashamed of." — *Sandra*

I was born in 1972, which meant I came of age in the 1980s. My family, like many, was tight-lipped about lots of issues, but especially those related to bodies or sexuality. There were certain things we just didn't talk about, period. My sisters and I, for example, did not use the anatomically correct words to describe our body parts. I honestly don't even know that our parents knew those terms. Instead, we relied on vague terms like "heiney" to refer to our buttocks and anything close to our anus. Interestingly, I have no memory of any term for vagina. As I grew older, went to college and ultimately had my own children, I felt it was important to make sure they had access to language and to accurate terms to describe their body parts. This was not always easy for me. I distinctly recall being in the supermarket around 2015 and my daughter yelling loudly: "This strap [in her stroller] is hurting my vagina!" Even though I had done my very best to ensure my children felt comfortable in their bodies, I blushed. I blushed at my daughter using an anatomically correct language to describe her body part because for whatever reasons at age thirty-six I still wasn't 100 percent comfortable with the term.

I share this story because I know many of you can relate to my experiences, or at a minimum, sympathize with them. There are many people walking around on the planet today who do not feel 100 percent comfortable talking about anything body or sex related. I get that—I really do! With that being said, in this section, I push on that thinking and encourage all of us to be open to new ways of thinking, talking and being in the world because I believe with all my heart that the health and well-being of millions of women depend on it.

The thing about silence is that it is usually a cover for shame. We often avoid talking about certain subjects because we've been told they're inappropriate or we've received an inaudible but strong message that those subjects are something to be embarrassed about. The most fascinating thing about shame is that it grows stronger the longer we stay silent. Before we know it, the way we operate in the world as people and the way industries like health care operate in the world are impacted by that silence. The silence I'm talking about results in:

- Girls feeling embarrassed when they get their first periods.

- Fewer clinical trials focused on women's health.

- Access to tampons and maxi pads being viewed as a woman's issue versus a health issue.

- Women "suffering" silently from perimenopause and menopause symptoms.

- Women and men worrying about telling their employer they will be out on family leave.

- Clinicians who don't feel equipped to have conversations with their patients about perimenopause or menopause.

All of this and more!

My chief goal in writing this guide is to give women the information they need to prepare for perimenopause. My secondary goal is to change how we think about, talk about and treat perimenopause. If I've learned anything in my lifetime it's that shame gets us nowhere. It prevents us from growing and evolving and in some cases, it can even prevent us from solving complex or serious problems. Colon cancer is a good example of this. Many people put off colon cancer screening or ignore the potential signs of colon cancer because they're too embarrassed to talk with their care team about their symptoms and too embarrassed to undergo the screening itself. According to the Centers for Disease Control (CDC), colon cancer is the third leading cause of cancer-related deaths in America. The third! People are literally and figuratively dying from embarrassment. It's clear we have some work to do. The first step in eliminating stigma is talking—talking about the things that may embarrass us. I say we start now by talking about perimenopause!

Talking about Perimenopause at Home

In talking with women about their perimenopause experiences many told me they weren't sure how to broach the subject with their families. They told me they didn't want to make a big deal out of perimenopause or worry anyone. I hear you and I'm not suggesting you set off a fire alarm every time you have a hot flash. Instead, here's what I recommend:

Talk with your partner, if you have one. Ideally, talk with your partner before you are in perimenopause. Choose a low-stress moment and casually ask them if they've heard of the term *perimenopause*. If they haven't, share what you've learned in this guide. Stick with the big picture and reassure them perimenopause is a natural process. Explain you've read this guide because you want to be knowledgeable and prepared for whatever you may experience. If it feels right to you, let them know that you will be tracking your symptoms and invite them to share anything they notice about your emotional or physical health. If you have experienced mental health issues in the past, explain to your partner you're at greater risk for mental health issues during perimenopause and enlist their support in tracking your well-being. You may also want to discuss treatment options with your partner ahead of time and discuss with them any questions or concerns they may have. The reality is that many treatment options affect our partners, even if it's just a finance issue, so it's best to get on the same page. With that said, it's your body and I encourage you to make decisions you believe will work best for *your* body.

The most important reasons to talk with your partner about perimenopause are for support and to normalize this health stage of life. If you do struggle with challenging symptoms or need to treat multiple symptoms, you will want your partner to be at the ready to support you. I was so busy being superwoman when perimenopause hit that my partner was suddenly thrust into taking on more responsibility at home because I was not able to function as I once had. Looking back, I wish I had given him a sense of what to expect so he could have been prepared to support me. Talking with your partner is one way of expanding the anti-stigma effect. If we all talk with our partners, give them accurate information, and normalize the perimenopause process they won't feel like perimenopause is something to worry about or fear and they will be able to speak freely about it with their friends and others. Additionally, research shows when partners are knowledgeable about these issues, women's quality of life improves.[77]

It's never too late to talk with your partner. You may be in perimenopause as you read this guide and you haven't yet had a conversation with your partner. It's not too late! I was about midway through perimenopause when I began to understand what was going on. When I clued in my partner he was incredibly relieved to have some answers as to why my health and happiness had plummeted so badly. He had been worried and frustrated and felt helpless until he had a name to go along with what I was experiencing. Once he knew what we were dealing with he had lots of questions and frankly he also had a lot of misconceptions and stereotypes rolling around in his brain. Our conversations were an opportunity to give him accurate information and dispel those stereotypes. I remember vividly him saying at one point: "Everything I've seen on TV or in movies has made perimenopause sound like something I should fear. Like maybe you would become mean and nasty to me. I wonder why it's portrayed that way?" Given

77 Bahri N, Yoshany N, Morowatisharifabad MA, Noghabi AD, Sajjadi M. The effects of menopausal health training for spouses on women's quality of life during menopause transitional period. Menopause. 2016 Feb;23(2):183–188. doi: 10.1097/GME.0000000000000588. PMID: 26783984.

that it was only a couple decades ago that menopause was described in books as "a serious, painful, and often crippling disease," it's not surprising those sentiments are still in some of our mindsets.

Talk with your children, if you have them, or nieces, nephews etc. If we're going to normalize perimenopause and lift the stigma of this natural stage of life, we need to give the next generation accurate information and be open and honest about this phase of life. This kind of conversation may be hard for you or for your family if you don't typically talk about topics like this. Go at your own pace and at your and their comfort levels. I have been very matter-of-fact with my teenagers as I've been writing this guide, saying things like: "Perimenopause is a stage most women go through in their early forties to early fifties. It means my hormones are changing, but there's nothing to worry about. I'm tracking my symptoms and working with my doctor to treat any symptoms that interfere with my life."

Notice how I am suggesting talking with your children, not just your daughters. I truly believe the subject of perimenopause won't been seen as a normal stage of life until all genders view it and treat it as so. Being open and honest with your children of all identities is key to changing the stigma.

Talk with your mother and female relatives. As I've spoken with women who are a generation older than me, I've developed deep empathy for their experiences. They've lived through the stigma I'm committed to ending and they've lived to tell the story. Sadly, my sense is that they have never actually had an opportunity to share their stories even in their own families. I'm not suggesting you ask your older female relatives to put on a perimenopause or menopause skit at your next holiday gathering. However, you may want to ask them what their experience was like, how they coped, what treatments, if any, worked for their symptoms and what they wished they had known prior to perimenopause. To eliminate shame we need to give those who have felt shame an opportunity to share their experiences should they wish to.

Talk with all of your clinicians. I discussed in detail in Chapter 8 the importance of creating a perimenopause dream team, but I also encourage you to tell any other clinicians you see three things:

1. That you are currently in perimenopause (or tell them you believe you are approaching perimenopause if you are not there yet and ask for their advice on how to prepare).

2. Any symptoms you're experiencing.

3. All treatments you are taking for your symptoms, including integrative treatments like herbs and acupuncture.

I encourage this kind of transparency for two reasons. First, our health-care system is not as coordinated as would be ideal. Even with the increase of electronic medical records, many of our clinicians have no way of knowing what kind of treatment we receive outside their offices. You want to make sure they are fully aware of all treatments and medicines so they don't prescribe or treat you in any ways that will interfere with your perimenopause care. Second, as I'm sure I've made crystal clear in so many ways throughout this guide, perimenopause is a sidelined health phase/condition. We can all help the health-care profession evolve by being open and unembarrassed about this stage of life and normalize talking about it and seeking treatment when needed. My greatest hope is once the health-care industry fully understands that each day six thousand women reach menopause our care will become a priority.

Talk with your colleagues. Women over fifty are one of the fast-est-growing demographics in the workplace. The US Bureau of Labor Statistics estimates there will be more than 55.1 million women fif-ty-five and older in the US labor force by 2024.[78] As a result, many of us will go through perimenopause and menopause while working and trying to advance our careers. This can get tricky if we experience significant symptoms that interfere with our lives. As I shared earlier in this guide, I sat down with my two business partners at one point in perimenopause because I was barely able to get out of bed let alone perform my work functions to my usual level. I explained I was con-cerned about my symptoms and I reassured them I was doing every-thing in my power to get to a better place physically and emotionally. You may not have a close relationship with any of your colleagues or feel comfortable sharing health information with them and in that case, there's no reason to. However, if you trust your colleagues and you have a good relationship with them, I encourage you to be open even if with just one colleague just as you would if you were struggling with a health condition of any other kind. If you prefer, you don't even have to share the specifics about perimenopause but I encourage you to say something like: "I'm dealing with some health issues right now and it's been a challenge. I'm working with my doctor/clinician/care team to manage things." I recommend being open because we need support when we're dealing with health challenges and pretending like nothing is wrong does no one a service.

> **IMPORTANT NOTE:** As of winter 2021 as I write this guide, perimenopause and menopause are not considered a disability under the Americans with Disabilities Act. This is the case even

---

78   www.bls.gov/opub/mlr/2015/article/labor-force-projections-to-2024.htm

though up to 75 percent of women in menopause experience vasomotor symptoms and others experience insomnia, mood swings brain fog and more, all of which may interfere with their ability to perform their job duties. Members of Parliament in the United Kingdom have introduced legislation to recognize and protect working women going through the challenges of menopause by requiring employers to make accommodations for them, such as through flexible working policies. If the legislation passes, it may turn the tide in the United States and other countries. Until then, I advise all women to be careful about disclosing anything related to perimenopause and menopause to their employers.

A FINAL WORD

This whole chapter is about ending stigmas, normalizing women's health issues, raising awareness, changing the health care system and talking about perimenopause—to anyone and everyone. With that said, if you aren't comfortable doing any of those things, I totally and completely get it. Our journeys don't have to be identical or even similar. If you picked up this guide to find one or two ways to make this time of life more manageable and that's it: more power to you. And, if you *are* the person who has been trying to find ways to talk with the people you love or your care team about your perimenopause experience I hope this chapter affirms that goal and gives you ideas for how to begin those conversations. All my best to *both* of you.

Chapter 17:

HIGHLIGHTS AND WHAT'S NEXT?

Here you are, at the end of this book. So what have we learned? Here are some highlights:

- Perimenopause is a natural stage of life that lasts on average four years but can last as long as ten to fifteen years.

- Some women sail through perimenopause, but the majority of us experience physical and emotional symptoms, many of which are challenging.

- Some of us experience a double whammy and get a thyroid diagnosis during perimenopause, which can complicate things.

- Thyroid disease is a hidden epidemic among women and you need to understand how your thyroid works and what your body needs. You will need to advocate for yourself to get the care you need and deserve.

- Unfortunately, most health-care clinicians are not trained in women's reproductive health and sexual issues, including hormone balancing, perimenopause or menopause.

- We all deserve a perimenopause dream team with deep expertise in hormone balancing.

- Testing our hormones often is important.

- If you have struggled with PMS, depression, anxiety, bipolar or other mental health issues prior to perimenopause, be on the lookout for those symptoms to return or exacerbate in perimenopause. Work with a mental health professional and care team with expertise in hormone balancing.

- Despite the lack of available information, HRT is a viable option for many of us.

- There are lots of things we can do to positively impact our perimenopause journey including getting good sleep, moving our bodies, eating for hormone health and limiting alcohol.

- Stress does a serious number on our hormones. Find ways to limit stress—please!

- Herbal remedies help some women, including me, and could help you. Do your research and work with your health care team.

- Perimenopause does not mean we are old, dried up and at the end of our lives. It can be a jumping-off point to a new and exciting stage of life.

- We can all play a part in ending the stigma associated with women's reproductive health, including perimenopause. The first step is talking without shame with our friends and family members.

So, what's next? I hope you'll join me at Periwinkle (www.helloper-iwinkle.com) where we will continue the conversation, support one another and go deeper into whatever topics interest you most about thriving in midlife.

And, finally, a request to you dear reader: if you have enjoyed this book and if you have found it informative, please go to **Amazon** and **Goodreads** and leave me a review. The challenge with perimenopause is that there isn't enough information available that is easy to read and understand and my hope is that this book fills that gap. Algorithms, however, rule the world these days, which means books without reviews are not advertised by Amazon or other booksellers. Reviews (not just star ratings) make all the difference. I know you're busy but even just a "Really liked this book. The information has helped me with Perimenopause" or something like that would be helpful. Thank you, Thank you, Thank you!

ACKNOWLEDGMENTS

Thank you to the many women who shared their perimenopause and menopause stories with me. Thank you for being so open and honest.

I am very grateful to the pre-perimenopause women who so graciously and transparently shared with me what they need and want from a book about preparing for perimenopause.

I am grateful to the Arlington chapter of Moms Run This Town (MRTT) who first inspired me to write this book. Thank you and I hope this does the trick.

A huge thank you to Dr. Lakeischa McMillan, who is not only a caring, knowledgeable, and supportive clinician who helps women balance their hormones and manage thyroid disease, but she also kindly reviewed this book in order to ensure clinical accuracy.

I am eternally grateful to my friend and colleague Lois, who read first drafts of this book and shared constructive and supportive feedback on every page. You made this book better. Thank you!

Thank you to the Periwinkle Team, all of whom have been a joy to work with. You have understood my vision from day one and I appreciate each of you for the expertise you bring to our work.

I am always grateful to Christine and Colleen, my X4 Health cofounders for what we have created together. Thank you for enthusiastically encouraging me to take on this book and to launch Periwinkle. Impact is the name of our game—always.

I am incredibly grateful to my dear friends who listened to me talk about this book and about Periwinkle nonstop for many months. Thank for sharing in my excitement about shedding light on this important stage of women's lives, ending stigmas, improving health care and changing culture.

A special thank you to my family, who saw less of me as I holed myself away in my office to write and create for 8+ months and who cheered me on along the way. A very special thank you to Chuck for reminding me whenever I got exhausted or overwhelmed that, in my heart I am a writer and advocate for women. Thank you for seeing that writing this book and launching Periwinkle are my dream come true. Xoxo